Fella Benabed
Applied Global Health Humanities

Medical & Health Humanities

Aesthetics, Analyses, Approaches

Edited by
Mita Banerjee, Monika Pietrzak-Franger
and Anita Wohlmann

Advisory Board
Elisabeth Dietrich-Daum, Marie-Theres Federhofer, Arthur W. Frank,
Ericka Johnson, Erin Gentry Lamb, Jane Mcnaughton, Swarnalatha Rangarajan,
Heinz-Peter Schmiedebach, Jens Temmen, Kirsten Zeiler

Volume 4

Fella Benabed

Applied Global Health Humanities

Readings in the Global Anglophone Novel

DE GRUYTER

ISBN 978-3-11-139610-1
e-ISBN (PDF) 978-3-11-139639-2
e-ISBN (EPUB) 978-3-11-139658-3
ISSN 2940-9632

Library of Congress Control Number: 2024933455

Bibliographic information published by the Deutsche Nationalbibliothek
The Deutsche Nationalbibliothek lists this publication in the Deutsche Nationalbibliografie; detailed bibliographic data are available on the Internet at http://dnb.dnb.de.

© 2024 Walter de Gruyter GmbH, Berlin/Boston
Cover image: „Map of Health" by Odra Noel
Printing and binding: CPI books GmbH, Leck

www.degruyter.com

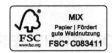

Preface

In founding the health humanities in 2006, I did not expect such a firework display of innovation to emerge worldwide in the mere eighteen years to the publication of this timely and compelling book by Fella Benabed. During that period, we have seen health humanities research units, projects, curricula, publications, conferences and impacts spread across all continents. Most importantly, we have witnessed how governments and policy makers have latched on to the significant contribution that cultural assets in the arts and humanities can make to healthcare, health and wellbeing.

In the rise of health humanities, we have seen a shift to what I have called elsewhere 'creative public health.' Creative public health is about taking seriously the ways that social and cultural assets outstrip centralised healthcare assets globally and thus can play a key role in protecting health and supporting the recovery of best possible lives despite the ravages of disease. Social and cultural assets scaffold identity, engagement, purpose and sociality; they directly and positively affect our bodies and subsumed minds.

Writing and reading literature is one of the most profound opportunities for humans to represent and explore human consciousness. In reading literature, we can consider and share time with diverse personalities, visions and drama co-created by authors and ourselves, journey into different kinds of thinking and emotion. We are not passive in reading. In a sense, all novels are co-authored. Together, writers and readers generate hallucinatory worlds. Every novel read is different, even with the same reader.

Novels and other works of literature share the foundation of storytelling and stories are humanity's greatest entry point to knowledge. We describe, invent and share our worlds through stories. Healthcare, health and wellbeing are dependent on stories to learn what things can help secure our futures, to provide those caring for us with insights into our lives and symptoms, and conversely for health practitioners to express what is happening to them and the environments they serve within. Without the mortar of stories, healthcare, health and wellbeing would lose context and direction for its scientific technologies and interventions. It would be inhumane and dehumanizing.

For far too long, of course, the Global North has dominated this currency of storytelling. In this volume, Benabed goes against the tide and enriches us with a glorious array of Anglophone literature relevant to health states in the Global South and multi-ethnic contexts of the Global North, focusing on the topical issues of infectious disease, mental disorder, disability and holistic healing. Her offering is important because health and wellbeing are ideally for everyone yet the political worlds we inhabit often limit who gets to be or remain physically and mentally well. Many accounts of health and wellbeing originate in the Global North and perseverate narrow, often culturally and geographically limited, perspectives on health, illness, and practices of cure and care. The experiences of and outlooks on health, illness, disease, disability and the broader notions of wellbeing or healing among those in the Global South and in multi-ethnic contexts in the Global North are less visible. This book offers visions for a future with more globally nuanced sensibilities and critical readings.

Professor Paul Crawford, University of Nottingham

Acknowledgments

I hereby extend my sincere gratitude to the persons and institutions whose support has played an essential role in the publication of this book. Foremost, I am indebted to the book series editors, Anita Wohlmann, Mita Banerjee, and Monika Pietrzak-Franger, whose trust and guidance have significantly contributed to the realization of this book. I also wish to express my acknowledgement to the anonymous reviewers whose valuable suggestions have considerably enhanced its quality and rigor. I would like to reserve a special acknowledgment for a distinguished figure in the field of global health humanities, Paul Crawford, for writing the preface and honoring the book with his expertise. I extend my gratitude to the Fulbright Commission that provided me with the opportunity to be a visiting scholar at Columbia University in the city of New York, along with access to its extensive library resources. I am particularly thankful to Rishi Goyal and Sarah Monks, from the Institute of Comparative Literature and Society, for facilitating this achievement. On a personal note, I am indebted to my father and husband, and especially to my late mother, whose encouragements have constituted the bedrock upon which my scholarly career has emerged. Lastly, I express my appreciation to my friends who have been a source of intellectual and emotional sustenance throughout this publication journey.

Contents

List of Figures —— XIII

List of Tables —— XIV

Introduction —— 1
    Applied Global Health Humanities: Bridging "the Two Cultures" —— 2
    Readings in the Global Anglophone Novel —— 6
    Research Questions and Book Structure —— 9

Part I: Global Health Humanities – Mapping the Terrain

1 Inclusivity in Global Health Humanities —— 17
    Introduction —— 17
    Definitions of Global Health —— 17
    Colonial History and Decolonial Ambitions in Global Health —— 19
    The Biopsychosocial Model of Global Health —— 26
    Medical/Health Humanities: Historical and Conceptual Underpinnings —— 27
    Inclusivity in Global Health Humanities —— 30
    Conclusion —— 38

2 Health Humanities and Global Anglophone Literature —— 39
    Introduction —— 39
    Literature and Medicine: A Time-honored Alliance —— 39
    Narrative Intersections of Literature and Medicine —— 41
    Ethical Intersections of Literature and Medicine —— 44
    Health and Well-being in Global Anglophone Literature —— 45
    Metaphoric Representations of the Diseased Body —— 48
    Metaphoric Representations of the Disabled Body —— 49
    Conclusion —— 56

Part II: Infectious Diseases in the Global Anglophone Novel

1. **Virgin Soil Epidemics and Unresolved Traumatic Grief in Louise Erdrich's *Tracks* —— 59**
   Introduction —— 59
   Virgin Soil Epidemics —— 59
   Unresolved Traumatic Grief —— 63
   Conclusion —— 64

2. **The Double Helix of Medical Knowledge Systems in Amitav Ghosh's *The Calcutta Chromosome: A Novel of Fevers, Delirium, and Discovery* —— 66**
   Introduction —— 66
   Ronald Ross: Figure of Scientific Imperialism —— 66
   Western vs. Occult Medical Knowledge —— 69
   The Double Helix of Knowledge Systems —— 71
   Conclusion —— 72

3. **AIDS: "Accelerated Inner Development Syndrome" in Meja Mwangi's *Crossroads: The Last Plague* —— 73**
   Introduction —— 73
   Reckless Responses to the Sweeping Epidemic —— 73
   Women's Vulnerability to the Epidemic —— 75
   Rational Responses to the Sweeping Epidemic —— 77
   Life Review and Accelerated Inner Development Syndrome (AIDS) —— 78
   Conclusion —— 81

Part III: Mental Disorders in the Global Anglophone Novel

1. **Lingering Wounds of Maternal Abandonment in Toni Morrison's *A Mercy* —— 85**
   Introduction —— 85
   The Trauma of Maternal Abandonment —— 85
   Mending the Mind within —— 88
   Conclusion —— 91

2. **Nervous Conditions in Tsitsi Dangarembga's Trilogy —— 92**
   Introduction —— 92
   Colonialist Conceptions of Nervous Conditions —— 92
   Nervous Conditions: Corporeal Resistance through Eating Disorders —— 94

The Book of Not: Corporeal Non-identity —— **97**
　　　Corporeal Grief in *This Mournable Body* —— **101**
　　　Conclusion —— **103**

3　Migration Trauma and Presenile Dementia in David Chariandy's
　　***Soucouyant* —— 104**
　　　Introduction —— **104**
　　　Intergenerational Transmission of Migration Trauma —— **104**
　　　Presenile Dementia as a Compounding Factor for Migration
　　　Trauma —— **108**
　　　Conclusion —— **110**

Part IV: Disability in the Global Anglophone Novel

1　Beyond "Narrative Prosthesis": Disability Interpretations in Bapsi Sidhwa's
　　***Cracking India* —— 113**
　　　Introduction —— **113**
　　　Game Plan of "Divide and Rule" —— **113**
　　　Literary Representations of Disability —— **115**
　　　Bharat Mata: The Embodiment of Motherhood and Victimhood —— **117**
　　　Conclusion —— **119**

2　Ableism and Disgrace in Salman Rushdie's *Shame* —— 120
　　　Introduction —— **120**
　　　Disability Models and Ableist Stereotypes —— **120**
　　　Intersections of "Narrative Prosthesis" and "Aesthetic
　　　Nervousness" —— **123**
　　　Conclusion —— **126**

3　"Aesthetic Nervousness" in John M. Coetzee's *Slow Man* —— 127
　　　Introduction —— **127**
　　　"Disability as Null Set and Moral Test" vs. *"Disability as the Interface with
　　　Otherness"* —— **127**
　　　Cure vs. Care —— **130**
　　　Conclusion —— **133**

Part V: Holistic Healing in the Global Anglophone Novel

1 **Autopathography and the Healing Garden in Bessie Head's *A Question of Power*** —— 137
   Introduction —— 137
   Autopathographic Exploration of Madness —— 137
   Cultivating Sanity in the Edenic Garden —— 139
   Conclusion —— 142

2 **Curative Eco-narrative in Leslie Marmon Silko's *Ceremony*** —— 143
   Introduction —— 143
   The Gynocratic Custody of Eco-healing Traditions —— 143
   The Etiology of Tayo's Illness —— 145
   Tayo's Ceremonial Rite of Eco-recovery —— 147
   Whole Again with the Human and the More-than-human Worlds —— 151
   Conclusion —— 152

3 **Eco-artistic Recovery in Delia Jarrett-Macauley's *Moses, Citizen and Me*** —— 153
   Introduction —— 153
   Child Soldiers' War Trauma —— 153
   Child Soldiers' Eco-artistic Recovery —— 156
   Child Soldiers' Rite of Passage in the Archetypal Forest —— 160
   Conclusion —— 162

Conclusion —— 163

Works Cited —— 169

Index of Persons —— 182

Index of Subjects —— 184

List of Figures

Figure 1: One Health
Figure 2: Robert Thom's Painting (circa 1952) "J. Marion Sims: Gynecologic Surgeon"
Figure 3: Representations of the Black Man in the Great Chain of Being
Figure 4: George Engel's Biopsychosocial Model of Healthcare
Figure 5: Nahuas Infected with Smallpox (16th century)
Figure 6: John Gast's "American Progress" as an Allegory of Manifest Destiny
Figure 7: Ojibwe *Midew* (Medicine Man) in a *Mide-wiigiwaam* (Medicine Lodge)
Figure 8: Ronald Ross and his Wife (1898)
Figure 9: The Double Helix
Figure 10: Slave Auction in the Deep South (circa 1850)
Figure 11: Station near Delhi (Partition of India, 1947)
Figure 12: Abanindranath Tagore's "Bharat Mata" (1905)
Figure 13: Maslow's Hierarchy of Needs
Figure 14: The Sweat Lodge Ceremony: Pre-Columbian Mesoamerican Temazcal

List of Tables

Table 1: Biomedicine vs. Ethnomedicine
Table 2: Ato Quayson's "Typology of Disability Representation"

Introduction

Global health humanities is a new realm of inquiry that is emerging at the intersection of global health and health humanities; this book is my humble contribution to the edifice through the lens of literature. As we observe the challenges of health and healthcare in the contemporary world, it is evident that a comprehensive understanding cannot be garnered from the sole perspective of the biomedical sciences. Starting from the premise that "Fiction reveals truths that reality obscures" (West 39), *Applied Global Health Humanities: Readings in the Global Anglophone Novel* aspires to be a thought-provoking book that invites readers on a journey through the many-sided terrain of global health humanities. I argue that global Anglophone literature has a role to play in shaping perceptions and responses to health-related concerns in the Global South, as well as among multiethnic groups in the Global North. I explore the historical, political, sociocultural, and ethical aspects of health in these locations by analyzing the complex questions of health, disease, and disability in a selection of global Anglophone novels. It is my conviction that global health humanities can contribute to the construction of more humane and equitable healthcare systems in which practitioners honor their consecrated bond and find the right balance between treating the body and soothing the mind.

In our human existence, few moments can rival the intensity of our encounter with healthcare professionals with whom our feelings fluctuate from the bottom of despair to the acme of hope. Accordingly, this book is inspired by my personal journey as a care seeker and caregiver[1]. I have learned about human fragility and resilience in the face of disease and death, as well as the power of empathy and communication in the healing process. My journey in the field of healthcare has at times been tarnished by the sense of pain and injustice in the face of unethical, indifferent, or mercenary physicians who embody the principle of "science without conscience."[2] Providentially, an eternal equilibrium is maintained in the scheme of life; whenever the darkness of evil prevails, there always looms the glowing light of goodness. My family and I had the chance to meet, in awe, with ethical healthcare providers who have comprehended the words of Sir William

---

1 I deliberately use the concepts of "care seeker," "caregiver," and "healthcare provider" throughout the book to emphasize their more inclusive and cooperative connotations in comparison to "patient" and "doctor."

2 "Science without conscience is the ruin of the Soul" [in French, "science sans conscience n'est que ruine de l'âme" (50)] is an oft-cited statement from François Rabelais' *Pantagruel* (1532). It suggests that scientific advancements, when devoid of a moral compass, can lead to the degradation of the individual, and by extension, to the degradation of the society.

Osler, considered the father of modern medicine, "The practice of medicine is an art, not a trade; a calling, not a business; a calling in which your heart will be exercised equally with your head" (368). They not only have the mastery of medical knowledge but also the art of empathy and communication. I have witnessed the transformative power of the compassionate look, the warm smile, and the gentle word of healthcare providers who take time to listen to their care seekers' worries and hopes, providing solace in the gravest times.

Applied Global Health Humanities: Bridging "the Two Cultures"

This book flows from my academic journey as a student and professor of literature with an entrenched passion for interdisciplinarity. I have specialized in the integration of postcolonial, ecological, and narrative approaches to explore the intersections of historical trauma and eco-healing patterns within scriptotherapeutic African and Native American novels. In so doing, I have unwittingly been rambling in the terrains of applied literature and global health humanities. The common thread of my research has been the effort to bridge what Charles P. Snow calls "the Two Cultures" whereby he argues that the sciences and the humanities often operate in mutually exclusive worlds with limited appreciation for each other's perspectives (169). Osler also notes, "the so-called Humanists have not enough Science, and Science sadly lacks the Humanities" (4). The chasm between them hinders the growth of a well-rounded knowledge and prevents the understanding of global issues.

Consequently, the choice of using the word "applied" before global health humanities in the title of this book is related to the field of "applied humanities" which appeared in the 1950s. The humanities departments around the world have been facing significant registration declines and substantial budget reductions. The decline in enrollment is probably not due to a lack of interest in humanities subjects, but rather to the students' loss of confidence in their potential to lead to attainable career prospects. Humanities courses are sometimes self-referential, meaning that they tend to analyze concepts, theories, or texts that are characteristic of the humanities disciplines themselves, without reference to other branches of knowledge or to the real world. Yet, there is a pressing need for the humanities to engage in meaningful discussions about their societal relevance, particularly in an epoch marked by artificial intelligence, virtual reality, and environmental issues. In his article entitled "Applied humanities," Erwin Steinberg observes, "One studies the humanities to gain useful knowledge about the world in which he lives, spiritual nourishment, and a sense of values" (442). Their interpretive aspect explores the essence of humanity, fostering both individual and collective self-awareness. Their study should be oriented towards the improvement of the human condition by leveraging the narrative competence, critical thinking, intercultural understanding, and civic engagement of students and professionals in all disciplines.

As an interdisciplinary field bridging medicine, humanities, and social sciences, medical or health humanities is increasingly recognized within healthcare practice and education worldwide, mainly in Anglophone countries of the Global North. Until now, however, it continues to be largely unfamiliar in my country, Algeria, where medical education is approached through the biomedical evidence-based model. It is one of my ambitions, through this book, to find a listening ear and bridge this gap; the aim is to introduce the field of global health humanities into the medical curriculum and play a role in the re-humanization of the discipline in my country and the Global South in general.

Even if health-related themes have often been treated in literature, there is a recent reflection on how literature is related to the broad concept of "Global Public Health" for a better appreciation of the way "discourse on health is transmitted across cultures" (Rose). This book hence addresses an important research gap in health humanities, related to global Anglophone literature, which requires significant scholarly attention. It covers a compilation of novels written by renowned Anglophone authors across diverse cultural contexts; each of them invites reflection on themes of disease and disability and their intersections with race, gender, class, colonialism, or migration. From powerful stories of resilience in the face of epidemics, to examinations of historical and cultural inducers of mental disorders, to explorations of holistic healing practices across cultures, the book aspires to offer a panoramic view of the diverse experiences that shape human understanding of health. The importance of the study, revealed through the literature review, lies in the scantiness of full-length books on the global Anglophone novel, or the postcolonial novel to use a more established concept, in relation to health humanities.

Despite the inclusive aspiration of health humanities, in reality, most literary studies related to health remain embedded in the Euro-American tradition, principally the English-speaking and mainstream tradition. In "Health and Medical Humanities in Global Health: From the Anglocentric to the Anthropocene," Claire Hooker et al. state that the domain of medical and health humanities has historically been associated with a Western perspectives. However, there is a discernible transition towards globalizing it. A major example is the World Universities Network Health Humanities Initiative (2021), where Scholars from around the globe gathered to claim this broader perspective. Prominent in their discussions is the integration of health humanities into health professions education across the world (203).

In exploring the expanding domain of health humanities, scholars underline the established supremacy of medicine. Presently, be that as it may, there is an emerging consensus that literary texts transcend being mere supplements to medical practice; they are increasingly recognized for their inherent value, serving as both supportive allies and autonomous entities. In "Health Humanities: The Future of Medical Humanities?" Paul Crawford et al. argue that "The very term 'medical humanities' encapsulates the dominant force in the discipline. Historically, medicine has captured the intellectual and clinical high ground" (6). Inherent in this book is the principle that literary texts are not only a "supportive friend" (Brody 1) or "disruptive teenager" (Macnaughton, "Medical Humanities" 927) to medicine, but they have an "intrinsic value in their own right" (Macnaughton, "The Humanities" 24). Preceding health humanities by the adjective "global" invests it with a more inclusive scope in the study of the global Anglophone novel. In "Introduction: Global Health Humanities and the Rise of Creative Public Health," Crawford further remarks that health humanities is maturing "as an energetic, robust, and inclusive field: one that signals a more co-created and co-operative vision for how the arts and humanities can stand as an interdisciplinary, and not solely medicalized, shadow health care service" (6). In this passage, the author signals the departure from a strictly medicalized approach and highlights the importance of an interdisciplinary one that integrates the humanities and the arts in the holistic study of health.

In "Global Health Humanities: Defining an Emerging Field," published in *The Lancet* in 2016, Kearsley A. Stewart and Kelley K. Swain define the essential skills healthcare professionals can hone in this expanding terrain. They say, "The core skills for global health practitioners do not focus on the doctor–patient dyad, but rather on understanding that the health of a patient is enmeshed in a complex system of individual behaviours, family and community relationships, environmental surroundings, economic limitations, and structural injustices" (2586). The authors provide examples of global health interventions inspired by the humanities, like Paul Farmer's *AIDS and Accusation: Haiti and the Geography of Blame* (1992). In this publication on the importance of storytelling in global health, the author traces the causes of AIDS to political history and globalization from the perspective of three Haitians. He contends that the proposition suggesting HIV originated in Haiti and disseminated to North America is rooted in racial and ethnocentric biases, lacking substantial evidence to support its claims.

Eve Darian-Smith and Phillip McCarthy propose a global methodological framework that offers the prospect of greater equity and inclusivity in knowledge formation. They argue that a "global imaginary" provides different perspectives on human actions and interactions that are not constrained by notions of "sovereignty, territoriality, citizenship, and nationalism." More importantly, it is an inclusive approach towards "non-Western worldviews, cosmologies, religions, aesthetics, ethics, values, ways of being and communicating, and perhaps even different ways of thinking about what it means to be 'human' " (4). Darian-Smith and McCarthy's global methodological framework, in which the influence of postcolonialism is noticeable, can be summarized as an inclusive approach that accepts multiple epistemologies beyond the worldview of the Global North. This holistic methodology analyzes interdependent societies and global-scale problems on a local-global continuum. It crosses North-South geographical boundaries, as well as temporal boundaries, to decenter knowledge production and dissemination. This approach involves historical contextualization that traces many aspects of present-day geopolitical cartography and global conflicts to colonial and imperial history. It involves the deconstruction of binaries like East/West, First World/Third World, and colonizer/colonized, recognizing the essential hybridity and fluidity that define global reality.

Along similar lines, the global turn in the humanities emphasizes the importance of non-Western cultures and their various forms of knowledge, enriching the traditional conception of the humanities by encouraging transcultural research. In his recent article, "From Global Studies to Global Humanities" (2023), Stefan Eklöf Amirell observes that in contradistinction to the development of global studies in the 21st century, there have been relatively few endeavors to establish global humanities as a field of study. He examines recent initiatives to advance it through the creation of scholarly communities, departments, and programs, as well as a few publications that delineate a research agenda for this field.

In their edited volume, *The Humanities between Global Integration and Cultural Diversity* (2016), Birgit Mersmann and Hans G. Kippenberg argue that the humanities need to be emancipated from the "colonial burden of Euro and West-centrism" and "move on to a condition of globality" (271). Pursuing a parallel argument, Lisa Lowe and Kris Manjapra bring their contribution to global humanities through the lens of postcolonial studies in an article entitled "Comparative Global Humanities after Man: Alternatives to the Coloniality of Knowledge" (2019). They criticize the history of "modern disciplinary knowledge formations," particularly the European monopolization of "the definition of the human" (23), and call for the decolonization of the humanities. They emphasize "the interdependence, relatedness, and coproduction of communities" (26), and advocate for an "analytic of relation" to "reckon with the coloniality of knowledge that divides and regiments the world into areas, objects, properties, and scales of meaning" (43). The implication is that non-Western perspectives on the humanities have long been marginalized, and that it would be useful to understand the mechanisms by which Western monopolization has influenced diverse cultures and societies. In these scant but important publications, the decolonization of the humanities is a powerful call for a more inclusive and diverse understanding of human experiences.

Readings in the Global Anglophone Novel

Considering this global turn in academia, *Applied Global Health Humanities: Readings in the Global Anglophone Novel* is historically contextualized by situating the authors in a slavery-colonialism-globalization continuum of struggles against oppression and discrimination in different parts of the world. Hence, postcolonialism serves as the most relevant theoretical framework because it examines the way colonial hegemony has enduringly affected the formerly colonized countries and their inhabitants by studying the themes of identity, hybridity, resistance, and so forth. Following Bill Ashcroft et al., the postcolonial theory can be used to study the locations and cultures "affected by the imperial process from the moment of colonization to the present day. This is because there is a continuity of preoccupations throughout the historical process initiated by European imperial aggression" (*The Empire* 2). This quote defines the spatiotemporal scope of postcolonial studies which addresses the impact of the imperial process from the time of colonization until the present day; it views that the concerns raised during the historical period of colonialism and imperialism continue to be relevant, notably in the context of globalization.

Postcolonial studies, therefore, encompasses the regions that have been impacted by European colonialism and imperialism in Africa, Asia, Australia, Latin America, and the Caribbean, as well as Indigenous, immigrant, and refugee communities in every part of the world. These regions and their populations have experienced varied forms of hegemony, ranging from settler colonialism, direct/indirect rule, internal colonialism, as well as all forms of economic and cultural dominance. For its broad spatiotemporal scope, therefore, the postcolonial theory is one of the most relevant critical tools for the study of the global Anglophone novel, with its underlying power dynamics and sociocultural issues. It recognizes the intersectionality of various forms of oppression based on race, gender, and class, in relation to health and healthcare. In this book, it is conducted in parallel with other theories of literary criticism like ecocriticism and ecofeminism, considering the importance of the environment for health and well-being.

While formulating the title, the conceptual choice shifted from the "postcolonial" novel to the "global Anglophone" novel, a choice that specialist have recently made to name the literary works written in English throughout the globe. Because the concepts of "postcolonial" and "global Anglophone" are not mutually exclusive, I have made the choice of adopting the global dimension regarding the geographical and ideological scope of the book while maintaining the postcolonial theory as a major framework of literary analysis. Another reason underlying the lexical choice of "global Anglophone" is that "postcolonial" is increasingly being questioned. In the African and Asian contexts, some scholars argue that continuing discussions on the effects of colonialism may no longer be relevant, given that it formally concluded over sixty years ago. In the North American and Australian contexts, some others reject the theoretical framework because they conceal the colonial histories of the nations involved. In this manner, the use of "global Anglophone" is judicious to eschew similar disagreements. It includes literary works written in English, originating not only from former British colonies but also from nations without British colonial legacies. Additionally, it encompasses countries whose postcolonial identities might not be officially recognized.

The concept of "global Anglophone" initially appeared as "World Anglophone" in a 2018 special edition of *Interventions: International Journal of Postcolonial Studies* entitled "From Postcolonial to World Anglophone: South Asia as Test Case." This special edition "brings the U.S., Canada, Australia, and Ireland back into the fold without automatically necessitating an anticolonial perspective" (Srinivasan 310). The same journal has recently issued a 2023 special edition in which the term "global" replaces "world" in line with the global turn in academia. The aim is "to broaden the conversation by incorporating scholars with expertise in other literary and cultural traditions in the English-speaking world – Africanists, Caribbeanists, and Ethnic Studies scholars, as well as those trained in the more 'traditional' fields of British and American literature" (Lawrence 2). In an infinitely intertwined world, this inclusive approach reflects the polyphonic concert of cultures from diverse geographical areas.

While accepting that literary works have an intrinsic esthetic value that needs to be studied per se, this book rests on the belief that "literature does not float above the material world in some aesthetic ether, but, rather, plays a part in an immensely complex global system" (Glotfelty xvii). Consequently, the focus is on the concrete, real-world concerns that need to be at the heart of applied literary studies, keeping with the trend towards effect-driven research and practice, geared toward individual and societal benefit. As early as 1920, George Howe observed, "We are familiar with the distinction in the realm of scientific study between pure science and applied science. May we not apply the same terms to literature, and recognize the distinction between pure literature and applied literature?" (437). The distinction between pure science and applied science is commonly accepted, but the distinction between pure literature and applied literature, or literature in practice, is less commonly known. In fact, in its essence, literature has the ability to evoke emotions and provoke thoughts on the human condition, inviting immediate applicability in the social terrain. In "Applied Literature," Crawford et al. explain:

Literature – both fiction in a range of forms and autobiographical narratives, including pathographies – can tell us not only about medicine or doctors, but also about the experience of health, sickness, illness, encounters with clinics and clinicians, the reactions of significant others, the support found in the strangest of places, the role and impact of informal caring, and the radical reordering necessary after the dramatic rift that significant illness causes through an individual life. (38)

The quote is relevant for this study because it introduces the concept of "applied literature" in health humanities. It shows that literature goes beyond providing information about medicine or physicians; it explores the humane aspects of disease and disability, including the perspective of the care seekers, the support they receive, and the impacts their health conditions have on their lives.

It is from the preceding importance of "applied literature" that I use the concept of "applied global health humanities" in the title of this book. This choice aims to go beyond the purely biomedical aspects of global health and consider the cultural, social, economic, and political factors that influence health outcomes. The term "applied" suggests that insights from the humanities, and literature in particular, can be actively used to inform and improve practical aspects of global health. By engaging with global Anglophone novels on disease and disability, readers gain access to diverse perspectives and emotions related to health and healthcare in different cultures. These novels become a medium through which readers can understand the nature of personal experiences, along the historical, political, and sociocultural conditions underlying global health.

The novel is a particularly suitable medium for studying the intersection between literature and global health. Unlike other genres, it provides space for detailed character delineation and narrative structure, allowing writers to depict the physical, psychological, and sociocultural dimensions of disease and disability; it equally prompts readers to immerse into a versatile experience. Compared to ethics cases and case histories used by healthcare students and professionals, the long form of the novel provides room for broad contextualization and allows the exploration of ethical dilemmas in healthcare. The choice of the novel also comes from its prominent importance in postcolonial studies, as it is the essential vehicle to understand the reality of the nation, and the master tool of criticism and subversion of hegemonic master narratives. Its importance is further due to its accessibility, as it uses a language that is more explicit than the language of poetry. More importantly, it is more available and convenient for reading, especially at the time of e-books, compared to drama that is performed, noting that theaters are not widely available in countries struggling with socioeconomic challenges.

The global Anglophone novel is the space of cross-cultural expression par excellence as it reflects the experiences and values of the community in which it was written; it is often situated in a specific historical context that makes it useful for exploring the long-term effects of slavery, colonialism, or migration on the individual and society. It is multivoiced as its sophisticated narrative structure accommodates varied voices, including marginalized ones. It is useful to explore the relationships between the slaveholder and the slave, the colonizer and the colonized, the native and the immigrant, and many other power-based relationships. The subgenre of autofiction is particularly relevant for this study, as many of the selected authors blur the boundaries between fact and fiction to probe into their personal experiences with disease and disability, exploring the connections between individual stories and larger sociocultural, historical, and political narratives.

Research Questions and Book Structure

To orient my analysis of diverse Anglophone novels written in various regions of the world, I have sought answers to the following questions: How does the book bridge disciplinary boundaries between global health and the humanities? How can the global Anglophone novel contribute to the field of global health humanities? What are the key novels and themes that can better represent this emerging field? How do the authors explore the relationship between disease, disability, health, history, culture, and society? How do the selected novels depict the lived experiences of individuals and communities affected by global health disparities? What role does literature play in raising awareness and promoting empathy for people suffering from disease or disability? Engaging with these questions has the potential to enhance comprehension of global Anglophone literature in relation to disease, disability, health, and well-being. To answer them, I rely on close reading and textual analysis that allow a careful examination of the selected novels, employing literary analysis to highlight characterization, metaphors, symbols, and other stylistic devices that serve the themes of disease and disability. In parallel, I have recourse to historical contextualization because the global Anglophone novel is deeply invested in historical considerations related to slavery, colonialism, and migration, as well as sociocultural considerations related to race, gender, and class. This literary study is inherently interdisciplinary, drawing from diverse fields such as global health, the humanities and the social sciences to foster a cross-fertilized discussion of the selected novels.

The book is divided into five parts. The first historico-theoretical one maps the terrain of global health humanities in general, and in relation to literature in particular. The four following parts illustrate the concept of applied literature by analyzing specific global Anglophone novels on disease and disability across a wide geographical spectrum. The study encompasses novels written by twelve authors, seven females and five males, published between 1973 and 2018. Most of them are seminal authors who have contributed to the formation of the postcolonial canon, but some of them are lesser-known authors whose vivid writing is expanding the canon of what is now being renamed "the global Anglophone novel." The selection rests on the relevance of these novels, as they directly address a wide thematic range related to infectious diseases, mental disorders, cognitive or physical disabilities, and holistic healing, with significant intersections among these themes. The selection also rests on diverse geographic representations that permit a broader exploration of disease and disability on a global scale, within specific historical and cultural contexts. The selected novels have scholarly merit in terms of literary quality, cultural insight, and critical perspective; they are written by authors with an established literary reputation.

Part I, "Global Health Humanities: Mapping the Terrain," calls upon readers to participate in an interdisciplinary exploration of the maturing field. It provides a historical and theoretical contextualization for the book, an overview of the key concepts, theories, and methodologies that shape the intersection of the humanities and global health. It highlights the essential role of literature in general, and global Anglophone literature in particular, in understanding the connections between global health and human experience, with a broad comprehension of the historical, sociocultural, and ethical dimensions of disease and disability. It refers to the historical linkage between colonialism and medicine, with the related fields of postcolonial trauma studies and postcolonial disability studies. In so doing, the book foregrounds its contribution to the advancement of global health humanities.

Chapter One, "Inclusivity in Global Health Humanities," sheds light on interrelated factors such as race, gender, and class as social determinants of health, and their effects on the individual's experience of disease and disability. By expounding the colonial history of global health, as well as the growing decolonial approach towards it, this chapter calls attention to the role of global health humanities in addressing health disparities and fostering more inclusive and equitable healthcare practices across the world. Chapter Two, "Health Humanities and Global Anglophone Literature," starts with the exploration of the age-long alliance between literature and medicine before moving to the importance of a more inclusive approach that takes into consideration global Anglophone contributions. It emphasizes the importance of literary works from diverse cultural backgrounds in the understanding of disease, disability, health, healthcare, and well-being on a global scale.

Part II, "Infectious Diseases in the Global Anglophone Novel," concentrates on three novels that deal with infectious diseases in different historical and sociocultural contexts; it shows the relationship between disease outbreaks, human behaviors, societal responses, and health disparities. Through the selected novels, this part illustrates the connections between colonialism and tropical medicine and sheds light on the manipulation of medical knowledge by imperial powers. Embedded in the characters' quests for truth and knowledge, therefore, is the authors' ability to intertwine medical knowledge with sociocultural critique.

Chapter One, "Virgin Soil Epidemics and Unresolved Traumatic Grief in Louise Erdrich's *Tracks*," explores the devastating impact of infectious diseases on the Native American community and the importance of Indigenous medicine. Through the study of historical trauma and cultural loss, it stresses the importance of incorporating diverse perspectives and alternative healing practices in the field of global health humanities. Chapter Two, "The Double Helix of Medical Knowledge Systems in Amitav Ghosh's *The Calcutta Chromosome: A Novel of Fevers, Delirium, and Discovery*," is about the malaria parasite in relation to colonial history and scientific discovery. Chapter Three, " 'Accelerated Inner Development Syndrome' in Meja Mwangi's *Crossroads: The Last Plague?*" explores the effect of the AIDS epidemic on a poor Kenyan village. It plays on the acronym "AIDS" to understand the psychological concept of "Accelerated Inner Development Syndrome (AIDS)" in relation to the medical concept of "Acquired Immunodeficiency Syndrome (AIDS)." The positive aspect of the tragic content lies in the potential of epidemics, and health issues in general, to catalyze personal growth and communal solidarity.

Part III, "Mental Disorders in the Global Anglophone Novel," examines the portrayal of psychiatric conditions, which also turn into disabilities when they limit the individual's inclusion in society, especially in many regions of the world with significant health disparities. The selected novels explore the difficulties faced by human beings who suffer from mental disorders as well as the social stigmas that surround their conditions. This part is particularly important in the context of postcolonial studies because formerly colonized countries have been home to some of the most atrocious human conflicts in human history, causing widespread nervous conditions among the populations. In "Colonial War and Mental Disorders," the final chapter of *The Wretched of the Earth*, Frantz Fanon claims: "The truth is that colonization, in its very essence, already appeared to be a great purveyor of psychiatric hospitals" (181). This passage reflects Fanon's thesis that the act of colonization, with its inherent violence, exploitation, and injustice, causes psychological trauma and distress.

Chapter One focuses on the "Lingering Wounds of Maternal Abandonment in Toni Morrison's *A Mercy*." Set in the late 17th century, it penetrates the lives and minds of multiethnic American characters who tussle with the residual traumas of maternal abandonment in the context of slavery, trying to unknot their narratives of pain, survival, and resilience. Chapter Two shifts to Zimbabwe to look into the topic of "Nervous Conditions in Tsitsi Dangarembga's Trilogy." Despite the number of years separating their publication, the three novels can better be understood when studied as a coherent whole to get the gist of the author's evolving consciousness on the nexus between colonialism, race, gender, and nervous conditions like traumatic stress and eating disorders. Chapter Three, "Migration Trauma and Presenile Dementia in David Chariandy's *Soucouyant*," probes into the narrator's life as he cares for his mother under the insidious progression of dementia. This medical condition is vividly portrayed in relation to migration and multiculturalism in Canada.

Part IV, devoted to the study of "Disability in the Global Anglophone Novel," goes beyond the conception of disability as just a metaphor or "narrative prosthesis" (Mitchell and Snyder 49) in literary works. In other words, disabilities are often employed primarily as symbolic devices or narrative tools rather than representing the lived experiences of people with disabilities, perpetuating stereotypes and stigmas surrounding their condition. Even though disability appears as a "narrative prosthesis" in some selected novels, an empathic reading underlines the representation of disability in ways that are more authentic. This part interrogates the historical, political, social, and economic configurations that affect the lives of persons with disabilities in different cultural contexts. It reveals overlapping concerns in disability studies and postcolonial studies regarding power dynamics, representation, and empowerment, seeking to challenge dominant narratives and advocate for social change. Despite the conceptual and theoretical connections between disability and postcolonial studies, there are not many publications on this intersection in the global Anglophone novel.

Chapter One, "Beyond 'Narrative Prosthesis': Disability Interpretations in Bapsi Sidhwa's *Cracking India*," examines the history of Indian Partition in relation to the dismembered body, in both its literal and metaphoric meanings, to denounce the disintegration of communities in the face of religious and political violence. Chapter Two, "Ableism and Disgrace in Salman Rushdie's *Shame*," reads into the allegorical and ableist representations of disability. Despite the author's use of disability as a "narrative prosthesis," i.e., a "crutch upon which literary narratives lean for the representational power, disruptive potentiality, and analytical insight" (Mitchell and Snyder 49), a more empathic reading reveals the social stereotypes that marginalize and dehumanize a person with a disability. Chapter Three, "'Aesthetic Nervousness' in John M. Coetzee's *Slow Man*," revolves around a middle-aged Australian whose leg is amputated in a bicycle accident, leaving him dependent on other people's care. Using Ato Quayson's concepts of "aesthetic nervousness" and "typology of disability representation," the chapter illustrates the relevance of type 1, "*Disability as null set and/or moral test*" (37) and type 2, "*Disability as the interface with otherness*" (37).

The book ends in Part V with the exploration of "Holistic Healing in the Global Anglophone Novel." With full appreciation of the progress and performance of biomedicine, this part uses three global Anglophone novels to focus on the importance of integrative therapies that contribute to human health and well-being. In these novels, nature is a centerpiece in the holistic healing process of the ailing characters who suffer from mental and psychosomatic disorders; their recovery is approached through alternative treatments like forest therapy, garden therapy, art therapy, and eco-artistic recovery. This part concludes with the global environmental health humanities approach that broadens the horizons of the growing discipline. Integrating a green dimension highlights the impact of environmental degradation on human health, prompting critical discussions toward environmental sustainability and planetary health. In addition to encouraging reflection on the environmental determinants of health, it promotes eco-consciousness and emphasizes the therapeutic benefits of nature in healing processes.

In Chapter One, "Autopathography and the Healing Garden in Bessie Head's *A Question of Power*," the study reflects the sociohistorical conditions that drive the protagonist insane, as well as the communal garden cure that makes her whole again. In the context of apartheid-induced mental disorders in South Africa, farming takes on spiritual and transcendental dimensions that allow agency and resilience. Chapter Two, "Curative Eco-narrative in Leslie Marmon Silko's *Ceremony*," reaffirms the healing power of nature in combination with the healing power of storytelling. Silko weaves a powerful curative eco-narrative to illustrate the importance of reconnection with the land and the community to heal the protagonist's Native American intergenerational trauma and WWII Post-Traumatic Stress Disorder. Chapter Three, "Eco-artistic Recovery in Delia Jarrett-Macauley's *Moses, Citizen and Me*," casts light on the transformative power of the natural environment and expressive art therapy in the rehabilitation of Sierra Leonean child soldiers. In a vision of communitas, the feeling of closeness among individuals who collectively undergo a liminal experience, the children recover their innocence in the same forest where they were bestially dehumanized.

From the applied literature perspective, the selected global Anglophone novels are valuable resources that offer alternative perspectives on human experiences of disease and disability, providing a tool for inclusive reading and attitudinal change. This approach of applied global health humanities acknowledges that novels about disease and disability are not isolated from the realities they seek to portray, but they are deeply embedded within them, shaping and being shaped by the web of interactions in global health.

Part I: **Global Health Humanities – Mapping the Terrain**

1 Inclusivity in Global Health Humanities

Introduction

Health humanities is an inclusive terrain characterized by interdisciplinarity and diversity; preceding it by the adjective "global" gives it a more inclusive scope and aligns it with the concept of global health. This chapter traces the history of global health to colonial medicine before moving to the decolonizing global health movement that promotes equitable healthcare across the world. This movement is in line with the essence of health humanities, an interdisciplinary terrain at the intersection of health and humanities disciplines, including medicine, philosophy, history, anthropology, literature, and the other arts, which has been expanding from the concept of medical humanities for more diversity, equity, and inclusion. The postcolonial, Indigenous, environmental, and feminist offshoots of health humanities highlight the intersectional nature of the involved disciplines, and the inclusive approach considers the various forms of discrimination, based on race, gender, and class that affect individuals and communities.

Definitions of Global Health

There is no consensual definition of the concept of global health, but for the purpose of this book, two definitions are worth noting. The first definition lists the six core principles of global health that are key concepts in the global Anglophone literary works to be later discussed in this book: "(1) cross-border/multilevel approach, (2) interdisciplinarity/transdisciplinarity, (3) systems thinking, (4) innovation, (5) sustainability and (6) human rights/equity" (Wernli et al. 010409). In this definition, the cross-border/multilevel approach emphasizes the need for international and interinstitutional collaboration. Interdisciplinarity and transdisciplinarity are essential to integrate diverse perspectives in addressing complex health challenges. Systems thinking recognizes the interconnectedness of Euro-America-centric and Indigenous knowledge systems. Innovation drives the development of novel solutions to address evolving health needs. Sustainability acknowledges the importance of long-term viability. Finally, the principles of human rights and equity advocate healthcare justice for all. Reading global Anglophone novels can contribute to satisfying the principles of global health in several ways. Firstly, these novels promote cross-border understanding by exploring diverse global cultures. Secondly, they integrate various fields of knowledge, enabling readers to develop an interdisciplinary understanding of health issues. Thirdly, these novels encourage systems thinking by depicting complex social relationships and knowledge systems. Furthermore, the diversity of Euro-America-centric and Indigenous knowledge systems can offer creative solutions to health challenges. They also address sustainability by showing the social, economic, and environmental factors that affect health. Lastly, these novels explore themes of human rights and justice, fostering empathy and empowering individuals to advocate for equitable healthcare systems.

The second definition of global health connects the health of human beings to the health of other-than-humans and the planet in the following words: "Global health, appropriately understood as an ecocentric concept, embraces the idea of healthy people on a healthy planet. This notion goes beyond anthropocentric considerations on health to include the importance of the interconnectedness of all life-forms and human well-being on an ecologically threatened planet" (Benatar 602). This conceptualization is in line with the concept of "One Health" that takes a comprehensive outlook on the interconnectedness between humans and other-than-humans, considering the health of all living beings and their ecosystems (see figure 1).

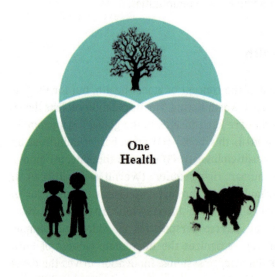

Figure 1: One Health (author's design)

The One Health Initiative Task Force of the American Veterinary Medical Association defines the concept of "One Health" as "the collaborative efforts of multiple disciplines working locally, nationally, and globally, to attain optimal health for people, animals, and our environment" (9). This imperative arises from the alarming degradation of the environment that is causing the proliferation of infectious diseases through viruses and bacteria, as well as non-infectious diseases through chemical contaminants.

The "One Health" approach aligns with the ethnomedical practices of Indigenous peoples, rooted in a sustainable relation to the land. In *All our Relations: Native Struggles for Land Rights and Life,* Native American environmental activist Winona LaDuke notes that "wherever Indigenous peoples still remain, there is also a corresponding enclave of biodiversity" (1). For instance, the Lakota phrase *"mitakuye oyasin,"* translated as "all my relations," is employed in healing ceremonies to reflect a holistic view of the web of life in which stars, planets, plants, and animals, are considered relatives (Modaff 341). In 1855, Chief Seattle proudly claimed, "every shining pine needle, every sandy shore, every mist in the dark woods, every clearing and humming insect is holy in the memory and experience of my people. The sap which courses through the trees carries the memories of the red man" (qtd. in Fahey and Armstrong 153–154). Therefore, the "One Health" approach holds significant importance to the green dimension of global health humanities adopted in the present study of global Anglophone novels with their intersectional examination of health, disease, and disability in relation to race, gender, and class.

Colonial History and Decolonial Ambitions in Global Health

The concept of global health was born of the need to find a more politically correct alternative to the concept of international health whose history is rooted in colonial tropical medicine (Koplan et al. 1993). There is, in fact, an increasing recognition that colonialism has left indelible imprints on medical knowledge and health systems. Scholars have recently been re-examining the resulting power dynamics and access to health disparities across the world. Throughout the history of global health, the relationship between race and science has influenced the health experiences of diverse populations worldwide. In *Fatal Invention: How Science, Politics, and Big Business Re-Create Race in the Twenty-First Century,* Dorothy Roberts argues, "Race is not a biological category that is politically charged. It is a political category that has been disguised as a biological one" (4); she adds that science was used as an instrument to give "the stamp of legitimacy" to racial difference (27). For instance, race-based medicine, in her view, "gives people a morally acceptable reason to hold on to their belief in intrinsic racial difference. They can now talk openly about natural distinctions between races – even their biological inferiority and superiority, at least when it comes to disease – without appearing racist" (167). In other words, while some diseases are affected by genetic factors, scientific research demonstrates, many diseases are determined or exacerbated by individual behaviors and socioeconomic conditions.[3]

During the slavery period in the United States, the need for dominance rested on racial stereotyping. In her revealing book, *Medical Apartheid: The Dark History of Medical Experimentation on Black Americans from Colonial Times to the Present*, Harriet A. Washington asserts that the dominance over blacks was reinforced by the 1840 census which linked black freedom with sexual promiscuity, disease (mainly syphilis) and contagion. This census presented slavery as necessary to maintain the health of blacks and protect whites from being contaminated. Medical journals diffused such data despite their fraudulent nature, demonstrating that manipulation of public health information was employed to advance a racist agenda (146–150). In addition, these unscientifically founded claims, along other myths like backs' alleged insensitivity to pain, intellectual slowness, and bodily uncleanliness, were used to validate unethical medical experiments. Involuntary sterilization, like the "Mississippi appendectomy" in the mid-20th Century, was widely practiced in the American South to prevent black women from frequent childbirth. This practice stemmed from racist ideologies that portrayed Black women as morally deficient because they had babies at a very early age. Daniel David Quillian reports in his article on "Racial Peculiarities: A Cause of the Prevalence of Syphilis in Negroes" that "Virtue in the negro race is like angels' visits – few and far between. In a practice of sixteen years I have never examined a virgin negro over fourteen years of age" (qtd. in Brandt 21). In his observation, the slavery supporting doctor does not admit the connection between early sexual activity and the sexual exploitation experienced by black girls.

Important artifacts and techniques used in modern medicine have been developed through morally questionable experiments based on racial domination. For instance, James Marion Sims, considered the "father of modern gynecology," developed medical and surgical instruments by brutalizing unanaesthetized African American slaves (see figure 2). This practice, which illustrates the claim of interracial difference in "pain thresholds," lies at "the very foundations of medical research itself" (DasGupta 35). Subjecting African American women to immense pain was based on the bias that different racial groups perceive pain differently, and it was only after years of experimenting on slaves that Sims treated white women (Jones 25). This kind of brutalization in the name of scientific progress remains a dark chapter in the history of medicine.

---

3 See David R. Williams' et al. "Race, Socioeconomic Status, and Health: Complexities, Ongoing Challenges, and Research Opportunities." *Annals of the New York Academy of Sciences*, vol. 1186, 2010, pp. 69–101. www.ncbi.nlm.nih.gov/pmc/articles/PMC3442603/

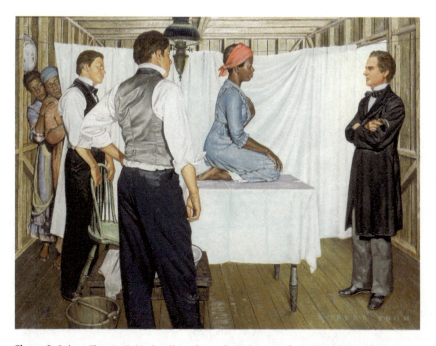

Figure 2: Robert Thom's "J. Marion Sims: Gynecologic Surgeon, from 'The History of Medicine'" (circa 1952), reproduced with permission from the University of Michigan Museum of Art Exchange. exchange.umma.umich.edu/resources/41241/view

Examining the historical trajectory of medicine, its role in slavery was comparable to its role in colonialism as a continuum of oppressive practices prevailed, and the medical authority was used to exert control over colonized populations. In his article, "Where is the Postcolonial History of Medicine?" (1998), Warwick Anderson asks this rhetorical question to emphasize the insufficient importance given to the role of medicine in colonial history. In reality, from the 17th century to almost the middle of the 20th century[4], scientific racism relied on racial differences to justify colonial expansion. In the "Great Chain of Being," the hierarchal order places the white man at the highest position and the black man at the lowest end of mankind, near the chimpanzee (see figure 3); Josiah C. Nott and Goerge R. Gliddon claim, "The palpable analogies and dissimilitudes between an inferior type of mankind and a superior type of monkey, require no comment" (547–548). The inferiority of some races was grounded on the pseudo-scientific arguments of phrenology,

---

[4] Scientific racism waned with the end of Nazism and WWII, particularly under the auspices of the UNESCO (Curtin 41–42).

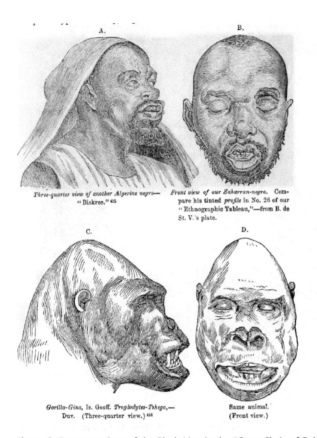

Figure 3: Representations of the Black Man in the "Great Chain of Being" (public domain image, Nott and Gliddon 548)

a practice that involved the study of the shape of human skulls to determine personality traits and mental faculties (Poskett 409). This laid the foundation for political aspirations at the heart of the global history of science.

In "The Construction of Racial Knowledge by Colonial Medicine in Africa," Delphine Peiretti-Courtis explains the mission of "bush doctors" to perform anthropometric research among Indigenous populations in the colonies, connecting their physical measures to their functional capacities. They not only sent survey reports to the colonial centers, but also human body parts. They conducted physiognomic research, judging the indigene's personality from their physical traits. They equally conducted inventories of African races, emphasizing aspects like the Bambara's "strength and docility" and the Wolof's "intelligence and obedience." These classifications, usually based on a "robustness index," served the different demands of the colonial workforce. The "pragmatic racialization of African populations by 'bush' practitioners," Peiretti-Courtis argues, "reveals the links between medicine, economics, and politics within a colonial context" (2). Hence, the "medical imperialism" (Schreier and Berger)[5] in the conception of the human was pivotal to the colonial enterprise of "civilizing mission" and the creation of white/black and civilized/barbarian binaries.

Colonial medicine considered primitivism as inherent to the construction of Indigenous populations; it advanced that their behaviors are controlled by their genes or some other bodily determinants. This biological deterministic view considered health issues as caused by their innate biological structure, insufficient hygiene, and rigid attachment to tradition. In its expansionist and hegemonic stance, therefore, imperialism associated "the power to govern" with "the power to heal" and relied on the assumption of "imperial cleanliness." Dominique Laporte contends:

If the history of modernity can be written as a triumph of cleanliness over bodily refuse, then so too could the European colonization of Africa and India. The sanitary crusade of the nineteenth century is central to the violent project of empire. Western medicine, with its emphasis on personal hygiene, functioned (and in some arenas still functions) as colonialism's benevolent cover. (37)

As stated in this quotation, colonial powers used hygiene as a justification for their presence and domination in conquered areas. They presented themselves as benevolent rulers who were bettering the life of Indigenous populations by highlighting their alleged superiority in cleanliness and healthcare. Despite the colonial presence for economic and political domination, this narrative functioned as a moral justification. It is important not to overlook, however, that many Western humanitarians genuinely valued public health and worked to lessen disease-related suffering. It is equally important to mention that Indigenous societies had their own healing approaches whose contribution to global health cannot be marginalized.

While discussing colonial medicine, Frantz Fanon's contribution cannot be underestimated, and his holistic conception of psychiatric treatment cannot be divided from the etiology of colonialist dehumanization.[6] His experience at the psychia-

---

5 See Herbert Schreier and Lawrence Berger's "On Medical Imperialism: A. Letter." *Lancet*, vol. 8, no. 1, 1975, p. 1161.
6 For his militant commitment against dehumanizing colonialism, Fanon can be regarded as an early champion of health humanities. His work was not recognized by the strictly biomedical system of his time he transgressed the boundaries between the sciences and the humanities. *Black Skin, White Masks* (1952), written in partial fulfilment of his psychiatric studies, was not accepted by the board of examiners for its references to politics, sociology, philosophy, and literature. "At that time and in that place," it was "altogether exceptional and atypical to see psychoanalysts pos-

try ward of Blida hospital in Algeria showed him the reality of the alleged "civilizing mission," causing him to resign from the workplace of "systematized de-humanization" (*A Dying* 53). He argues that "Western medical science" was one of the most "tragic" mediums of oppression because it was employed hand in hand with "racialism and humiliation" (*Black Skin* 121). It rested on the fallacies of scientific racism that affixed the native's behavior to a predetermined innate inferiority in brain structure. In the colony, Fanon argues, madness is predominantly "a pathology of freedom," adding that colonization, "in its very essence," is "a great purveyor of psychiatric hospitals" (*The Wretched* 181). Since mental illness is sociogenically constructed, he asserts, it requires a sociotherapy that takes into account the physical, sociocultural, and political aspects of disease.

Antoine Porot, considered the father of the Algiers school of psychiatry, provided a dismal picture of the native as genetically compulsive and aggressive. The Algiers school of psychiatry contended, according to Fanon, that a fully developed frontal cortex governed the Europeans' behavior while the diencephalon, "one of the most primitive parts of the brain," controlled the natives' behavior. The latter's cerebral constitution was allegedly to blame for their "mental and social inaptitude" as well as their "virtual animal impulsiveness" (*The Wretched* 225–227). This viewpoint highlights a problematic feature of colonial ideology, namely the use of racial and pseudoscientific beliefs to justifiably oppress and exploit colonized peoples. These disparaging presumptions about the social and mental abilities of the colonized were employed to maintain a sense of racial supremacy and support colonial hegemony. In turn, the English school of psychiatry, led by John Colin Carothers, submitted a report to the World Health Organization entitled "The African Mind in Health and Disease: A Study in Ethnopsychiatry" (1953). It presented adult Africans as children with excessive emotional lability and inability to mature, in a manner comparable to Europeans who were lobotomized, i.e., Europeans whose mental illness was treated by surgical incision of the frontal brain lobe.

Colonial psychiatry equally assumed that Africans "tended to be psychotic rather than neurotic, with a tendency towards schizophrenia rather than depressive disorders" while "manic-depression" required "a strong sense of personal responsibility, a quality originating in European culture" (Veit-Wild 13). This point of view is a reflection of the Eurocentric bias that existed in the psychiatric profession during colonial times. It is scientifically unethical because it negates the multi-

---

ing for themselves the political, ethnopsychoanalytic, and socio-institutional problem of their own practice" (Derrida 322). See Fella Benabed's "Fanonist Health Humanities." *Palgrave Encyclopedia of the Health Humanities.* Paul Crawford and Paul Kadetz, eds. Springer Nature, Palgrave Macmillan (forthcoming).

dimensionality of mental health that is influenced by biological, social, cultural, and environmental factors. Fanon argues that "science depoliticized, science in the service of man is often non-existent in the colonies" (*A Dying* 140). Medical practice and research, he claims, were affected by conflict of interest because the stakeholders were colonial landowners. Military physicians would violate medical confidentiality in defense of colonial power; they would denounce wounded combatants, abstain from treating them, and sometimes practice medically assisted torture to interrogate them. Fanon explains, "Everything – fear stimulant, massive doses of vitamins – is used before, during, and after the sessions to keep the nationalist hovering between life and death. Ten times the doctor intervenes, ten times he gives the prisoner back to the pack of torturers." If prisoners died, medical reports would specify "natural death," and if they did not, torture would put their "personality in shreds" (138). From these denunciations, Fanon's resistance against colonial medicine started; his decolonizing and re-humanizing approach to psychiatry is relevant for the current debates on global health and global health humanities.

Today, whatever the inclusive intentions at the heart of global health, scholars observe "colonial remnant" in some healthcare systems and practices to the point of claiming that "global health is old wine in a new bottle," and the decolonizing global health movement notes "many 'legacies' from the colonial times" (Kwete et al. 2). It adopts a postcolonial approach to reduce the hegemony of the Euro-Americans on the rest of the world in the field of healthcare. This hegemony looms large, for instance, in the context of pandemics in which healthcare systems in the North seek to dictate their policies on the South, usually blamed for the emergence of viruses. Much like tropical medicine that strove to protect colonizers from contagious diseases in remote outposts, some physicians seek international responses to HIV/AIDS, Ebola, and Covid-19 in Africa and Asia for fear of spreading them to the rest of the world. The process usually involves outspoken othering, hate speech, and sometimes violent attacks against Africans or Asians, such as the "Yellow Peril" stereotype about the Chinese. A major example lies in a TV comment made by Camille Locht, Research Director at the French National Institute of Health and Medical Research (INSERM), in which he suggested clinical trials of the BCG vaccine on Africans to prevent Covid-19 (Affun-Adegbulu and Adegbulu 2).

Even if the decolonizing global health movement has gained steam in the last few years, scant efforts in this perspective earlier existed. For instance, Alan Bleakley et al.'s article, "Thinking the Post-colonial in Medical Education" (2008), highlights the advantages of international partnerships in education, arguing that Euro-American medical curricula are often unquestionably adopted in the rest of the world. The authors believe that such practices might constitute a "new wave" of imperialism, and for this reason, a number of scholars are questioning them from a postcolonial perspective. In this sense, the suggested postcolonial/decolonial approach is useful to address the impact of colonialism on various aspects of global health. It calls attention to the unequal power dynamics inherent in global health systems that have practiced discrimination and contributed to the stigmatization and marginalization of populations in the Global South and ethnic minorities in the Global North.

The Biopsychosocial Model of Global Health

The need for a new paradigm of thought in global health finds expression in George Engel's biopsychosocial model introduced in his article, published in *Science*, "The Need for a New Medical model: A Challenge for Biomedicine" (1977). He cautions about the "crisis in the biomedical paradigm" that leaves "no room within its framework for the social, psychological and behavioural dimensions of illness" (129). He propounds the biopsychosocial model, connecting medicine to power and capital in the following words, "nothing will change unless and until those who control resources have the wisdom to venture off the beaten path of exclusive reliance on biomedicine as the only approach to health care" (135). Following this model, disease develops from the interplay between biological (genetic, biochemical, etc.), psychological (personality, behavior, etc.), and social (familial, economic, cultural, etc.) dimensions (see figure 4). For instance, despite possessing a genetic predisposition to depression, a person may not actually suffer from it without the effect of psychological elements like perfectionistic impulses as well as social factors like acute personal and professional stress.

Those in the medical community who want to infuse medical practice with more empathy and compassion find Engel's concept to be resonating. In 2002, the World Health Organization (WHO) decided to use it as the foundation for the International Classification of Function, Disability and Health (ICF). This approach is more important than ever at a time when science is transitioning from a purely analytical and specialized activity to one that is more holistic and interdisciplinary. In addition to being a scientific approach, it is also inherently humanistic because it deconstructs the Cartesian mind-body dualism, re-humanizes medicine, and empowers care seekers. The Covid-19 pandemic brought to light enormous healthcare disparities, making George Engel's 1977 biopsychosocial model of biomedicine even more relevant as it emphasizes that health is not just the absence of disease but also a state of total physical, mental, and social wellness.

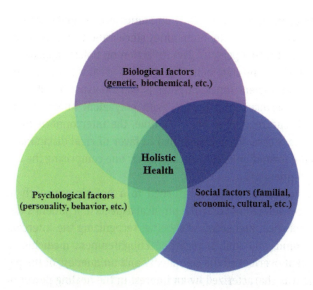

Figure 4: George Engel's Biopsychosocial Model of Medicine (author's design)

Medical / Health Humanities: Historical and Conceptual Underpinnings

The intersection of the humanities (philosophy, psychology, etc.), the social sciences (history, anthropology, sociology, etc.), the arts (literature, music, etc.), and their application to medical education and practice is where medical/health humanities comes into play. The discipline has emerged as a reaction to the mercantilization of medicine and the monopolization of techno-scientific knowledge, in an effort to foster "respect for individuals, protection of the vulnerable, tolerance of difference, care for those in need, equality of access, and the pursuit of justice" (Thomas Cole et al. 13). Neoliberal austerity measures have resulted in healthcare inequalities, stemming from the reduction of budgets and the commodification of services. The prioritization of profit and the commodification of medical treatment have resulted in the loss of empathy and the dehumanization of medicine. In this sense, medical/health humanities serves as an advocacy resource to humanize healthcare and challenge neoliberal austerity policies. It calls for a reflection on the human experience of illness, the sociocultural determinants of health, and the ethical considerations inherent to healthcare, emphasizing respect for individuals, protection of vulnerability, embrace of diversity, and pursuit of justice.

Even if the concepts of medical and health humanities are relatively recent, medicine has been in communion with the humanities since antiquity when it approached the care seeker as a whole person.[7] The reflection on holism appears in Aristotle's *Metaphysics*, to whom the statement "the whole is greater than the sum of its parts" is attributed. In ancient times, physicians were polymaths, like Ibn Sina (Avicenna), Nicolas Copernicus, and Galileo, with polyvalent knowledge in medicine, mathematics, literature, and so on. Over time, the interconnectedness of knowledge branches was progressively dismantled in favor of rigid disciplinary boundaries, resulting in the formation of two distinct blocs: one comprising the sciences and the other the humanities.

In the 19th century, Romantic medicine returned to a holistic approach to healthcare, as physicians considered not only the physical aspects of a patient's disease, but also their psychological and social well-being, recognizing the interconnectedness of the body, mind, and soul. It regarded Enlightenment medicine as being reductionist because it overlooked the complexity and uniqueness of the patient. Romantic medicine was characterized by an interest in the healing power of nature and the use of herbal remedies to promote health and well-being; it was also marked by the belief in the healing potential of arts, such as poetry, music, and painting. Yet again, by the early 20th century, medicine progressed considerably, leading to increased specialization, and physicians started dedicating their time to the command of a single branch of medicine. The Flexner Report (1910) geared medical education in American universities towards the biomedical model that gave priority to purely scientific knowledge, and critics of the reform apprehended that the humanistic role of medicine would be left behind. However, Abraham Flexner, the writer of the report, later regretted his choice, and in his *Medical Education* (1925), he wrote that medicine became "sadly deficient in cultural and philosophic background" (18). He confessed that the reform had transformed medical education into an aberration, leaving students with minimal opportunities for reading and contemplation. He expressed the need for more intellectual input and highlighted the value of the humanities in medical education to foster analytical thinking and humane intervention.

The concept of "medical humanities" first appeared in 1948 when George Sarton and Frances Siegel, commenting on the death of surgeon and educator Edmund Andrews, stated, "His death at the early age of 48 is a sad blow to the medical humanities" (127). The concept emerged amidst post-WWII debates on medical ethics, mainly related to the Nuremberg trials that disclosed Nazi physicians' experimen-

---

[7] In the Online Etymology Dictionary, "health" originates from the Old English word "hælan," meaning "to make whole" (Guidotti 189).

tation on humans. Medicine and the humanities had thus far been "entangled in a perverse love-hate relationship in which literature, history, and philosophy promised to soften medicine's rough edges." WWII reawakened the belief that the humanities "could nurture the soul of the doctor at a time when medicine, enraptured by science, was losing touch with the patient" (Wailoo 194–195). Unethical medical practices went on with the testing of new drugs without informed consent, such as the polio vaccine on children in psychiatric institutions (1950s) and the Tuskegee Study of Untreated Syphilis in the Negro Male (1932–1972). As such, scholars have realized that equipping medical students with necessary ethical and empathic skills through the study of the humanities is necessary to avoid similar malpractices.

The humanities have thence been considered as a remedy to "empathy decline," sometimes "moral erosion" and "clinical hypocompetence," among healthcare professionals (Platt 898) who can gain a deeper comprehension of the care seeker's suffering by reflecting on disease. This interdisciplinary approach combats the decline of empathy frequently linked to the demanding nature of clinical practice, as it fosters self-awareness, cultural competency, critical thinking, and humane healthcare. The 1980s witnessed the creation of medical humanities programs in numerous medical schools in the USA, partly due to the AIDS pandemic that brought to the fore non-biomedical debates on sex habits, condoms, and tolerance, "topics demanding integrated thinking about the human condition across the sciences, public health, social sciences, and humanities" (Wailoo 197). Scholars realized that evidence-based medicine is incapable of delivering the best quality healthcare without due attention to the humanities; they also understood the benefit of the humanities on the physicians' own well-being as they work in stressful, sometimes traumatic, situations.

In the last twenty years, critical medical humanities scholars have become skeptical of the consideration that the humanities are a "supportive friend" (Brody 1) or "disruptive teenager" (Macnaughton, "Medical Humanities" 927) to medicine. Jane MacNaughton asserts that the humanities have an "intrinsic value in their own right" ("The Humanities" 24) beyond the "use value" in the hands of humane physicians. The concept of health humanities, first used by Paul Crawford in 2006, thus emerged from the aforementioned argument that the humanities cannot just be medicine's "supportive friend" (Brody 1). It originated from the need to encompass other healthcare stakeholders formerly excluded from the discussions on medical humanities like nurses, social care workers, family caregivers, and the care seekers themselves. The discipline is presently prospering and actively incorporating various viewpoints and methodologies; as Craig M. Klugman and Erin G. Lamb observe, it increasingly "puts the humanities, arts, and social sciences in the center, rather than as an add-on to clinical and basic science" (3). It is not only concerned with conventional medical approaches, but also embraces interdisciplinary collaboration and draws on ideas from a variety of disciplines in the humanities.

Despite differences, the major similarity between medical and health humanities is that human disasters like wars and pandemics have played an important role in their development. In a manner reminiscent of how the AIDS crisis emphasized the significance of medical humanities during the 1980s and 1990s, Wailoo draws parallels with the global pandemic caused by the Covid-19 crisis. Marked by "underlying issues of disparate suffering, loss, blame, conflicted belief, social inequality, misinformation, and varied cultural responses," it has sparked renewed interest in health humanities (202). For instance, the sales of Albert Camus' *The Plague* (1947) soared, as it became the defining book of the global crisis. Set in the Algerian city of Oran, beleaguered by a terrifying epidemic, it provides a reflection on life and death, as well on the duties human beings have towards each other. Notably, it explores the altruistic self-negation and ethical responsibility of a physician in times of health crises.

Health humanities is growingly becoming a global, diverse, and inclusive field by borrowing theoretical concepts from the humanities like postcolonial, environmental, feminist, and disability studies. In Nehal El-Hadi's view, it is happening in three ways:

(1) by acknowledging and confronting the violently racist histories of medical and scientific knowledge; (2) by intentionally, deliberately, and carefully including works produced by racialized, marginalized, and oft-excluded individuals that explore narratives of the experiences of illness, disease, and the health-care encounter; and (3) by imagining possibilities for equitable health-care research, practices, and delivery. (43)

By confronting historical injustices, involving marginalized voices, and envisioning a more equitable future, health humanities can contribute to a transformative and inclusive healthcare system that serves all human beings.

Inclusivity in Global Health Humanities

Inclusivity is important for global health humanities because it ensures that diverse voices and experiences are represented. It recognizes that health issues affect communities and individuals in varied ways based on their intersecting identities, such as race, gender, and class. It emphasizes the interconnectedness of various forms of social oppression and discrimination to better address the health challenges faced by diverse populations. Inclusivity in global health humanities education can contribute to the training of culturally competent healthcare professionals who understand the diverse backgrounds and identities of their care seekers.

They can hence deliver a more effective and respectful care that leads to social justice and health equity for all humans. In this regard, the postcolonial theory provides a useful tool to adopt an inclusive approach to global health humanities that takes into consideration the relationship between health on the one hand, and imperialism, inequality, and oppression on the other, which still impact health and healthcare around the world. It explains that health, disease, and disability can be culturally constructed. For example, Indigenous healing practices, which are inherently holistic, may be considered by modern biomedicine as unscientific or even dangerous, but they can play an important role in promoting health and well-being in specific cultural contexts.

Indigenous health humanities is therefore another inclusive field that is gaining ground, recognizing the importance of ethnomedicine[8], the study of "different societies' notions of health and illness, including how people think and how people act about well-being and healing" (Quinlan 381). The role of ethnomedicine in the development of biomedicine is highlighted in the initial edition of the *U.S. Pharmacopeia* (1820) which contained comprehensive catalogs of 296 substances derived from animal, mineral, or plant sources, of which approximately 130 were Indigenous American medicinal remedies. The quantity of listed substances continued to rise in the *U.S. Pharmacopeia or the National Formulary* since 1888, categorized into anesthetics, narcotics, stimulants, astringents, cathartics, febrifuges, vermifuges, emetics, and more (Vogel 3). It is important, in this regard, to mention the notable recognition published on the website of US Embassy and Consulates in Italy in 2021, entitled "Native Americans' Many Contributions to Medicine," bringing into awareness that "Many of Native Americans' innovations in health and medicine have been around for thousands of years, predating – and contributing to – Western medicine." The website offers an example of chewed willow bark which contains an active ingredient, salicin, known for its analgesic properties. The origin of vaccines can also be traced back to Native American tribes that protected their bodies against the adverse effects of some substances by ingesting small quantities of them.

As it will be illustrated in two chapters of this book, Indigenous peoples suffer from intergenerational trauma that is vivid in their collective memory centuries after the settlement of Europeans. Maria Yellow Horse Brave Heart uses the concept of "Historical Trauma Response" (HTR) to designate the sense of loss that seems more deleterious than "Post-Traumatic Stress Disorder," as it is passed

---

8 According to data made public by the World Health Organization (WHO), in factsheet 134, ethnomedicine is still popular throughout the world, mainly in developing countries, but also increasingly in industrialized ones.

down from one generation to another (7). Consequently, many Indigenous persons express their grief by mutilating their bodies, drinking themselves into oblivion, sniffing glue or gasoline, and committing suicide or homicide (Wesley-Esquimaux and Smolewski 51). Historian Michael K. Smith writes, "They have twelve times the national incidence of malnutrition, nine times the rate of alcoholism, seven times the rate of infant mortality, five times the rate of exposure deaths, and several times the incidence of bubonic plague, tuberculosis, typhoid, diphtheria, and other easily preventable diseases" (369). Incapable of love, they also beat their partners, rape their children, and continually relive the violent past of their ancestors. Under oppressive conditions, ceremonial rituals allow Indigenous peoples to transmit oral traditions from one generation to another in the form of stories, prayers, and songs. Storytelling, in particular, offers a healing solution to the psychic wounds of individuals who need to tell their traumatic experiences, still vivid in the collective memory centuries after the colonization of their lands. It is usually an eco-narrative of healing that depicts ceremonies held in nature's passage from a season to another and an individual's passage from a phase of life to another.

In "Indigenous Health Humanities," Allison Crawford et al. study Indigenous life writing and artistic creations related to health. They identify four areas of investigation: "*1. Art and story as medicine,*" "*2. Art and story as knowledge and critique,*" "*3. Specificity, diversity and sovereignty of Indigenous knowledges,*" and "*4. Storytelling as relational—On being an ally reader/viewer/listener*" (101–102). Through these four areas, the authors shed light on Indigenous storytelling in the field of health humanities as an act of resistance against their exclusion and marginalization. Significantly, psychotherapist and storyteller Erica H. Meade enumerates thirteen features of stories that cure psychic diseases, but for the purpose of this literary study, it is useful to mention six relevant properties. Storytelling, according to her:

- Arouses strong emotions in the reader/listener,
- Presents people, situations, and actions that the reader/listener can identify with,
- Helps the reader/listener to externalize a conflict,
- Provides an opportunity for the reader/listener to draw healing by internalizing wise, helpful, or comforting figures in the story,
- Provides an opportunity for the reader/listener to model alternative attitudes and stances found within the story that can help when one is coping with hardship and trying to forge new paths,
- Helps people come to terms with duality, ambivalence, and strife, to move toward a more philosophical perspective on life. (243–247)

The cited properties present important arguments on the healing power of storytelling; the author shows that emotional engagement leads to the release of pent-up feelings through relatable characters and situations. She argues that a story can provide a mirror through which individuals can see themselves reflected, and the resulting identification is reassurance that they are not alone in their situation, no matter how arduous it might be. It also helps individuals externalize their conflicts by distancing themselves, understanding causes, reflecting on solutions, and learning lessons.

In "From the Clinical to the Ecocultural: Literature, Health, and Ethnoecomedicine," Animesh Roy coins the concept of "ethnoecomedicine" that reflects a holistic comprehension of health knowledge and its inseparable connection with natural resources within indigenous communities (252). In this regard, to understand the Native American novels selected in this study, the comparison between biomedicine and ethnomedicine is productive in terms of underlying principles, cultural groundings, disease causes, approaches to treatment, healthcare provider, healthcare recipient, and healthcare setting (see table 1). It is essential to note that these are not absolute distinctions because many healthcare systems and physicians' personal initiatives incorporate elements from both approaches to provide a holistic and culturally sensitive treatment centered on the care seeker.

Table 1: Biomedicine vs. Ethnomedicine

	Biomedicine	**Ethnomedicine**
Underlying principles	It is a scientific approach based on the principles of empirical research, clinical trial, and evidence-based practice. It is transmitted through Western-model education.	It is based on a holistic approach rooted in Indigenous knowledge and belief systems. It is transmitted from one generation to the next by word of mouth.
Cultural groundings	It emphasizes the universality of healthcare based on Euro-American biomedicine, regardless of cultural specificities.	It is deeply rooted in specific ceremonial rituals that vary from one ethnic group to another.
Disease causes	It posits that diseases are caused by specific physiological factors such as genetic variables, anatomical abnormalities, biochemical imbalances, and environmental factors.	In addition to physiological factors, it argues that diseases are caused by an unbalance between the body, mind, and soul, in relation to community and nature.
Approaches to treatment	It follows standardized protocols and guidelines, including specific testing and screening, pharmaceutical drugs, medico-	It uses herbal remedies and ritual ceremonies to address the many-sided aspects of health and well-being like Chinese acu-

Table 1: Biomedicine vs. Ethnomedicine *(Continued)*

	Biomedicine	Ethnomedicine
	surgical procedures, medical devices and therapies based on scientific research and clinical trials.	puncture, Islamic cupping therapy, and Indian Ayurveda.
Healthcare provider	The healthcare provider is a physician or medical professional who received formal education and training in Euro-American medical practices, acquiring an authoritative role in the healthcare process.	The healthcare provider is a community member – called Indigenous healer, shaman, herbalist, or medicine man/woman – who inherited or acquired the healing skills through communal apprenticeship, oral tradition, and spiritual guidance.
Healthcare recipient	The healthcare recipient, referred to as patient, is often considered as a passive receiver of medical care despite scientific evidence on the necessity of giving them a more active role (on the evolution being made in this regard, see Szasz and Hollender's contribution below).	The healthcare recipient, referred to as health seeker or care seeker, is engaged in active collaboration with the healer by making lifestyle changes, following ceremonial rituals and symbolic practices.
Healthcare setting	It usually happens in a healthcare facility (clinic, hospital), or at home, depending on the need for inpatient or outpatient care. Despite scientific evidence on the benefit of healing environments, healthcare usually happens in cold white-walled settings with no view on nature (on the evolution being made in this regard, see Ulrich below).	It sometimes happens at home or in a healing lodge, but more frequently outdoors, as in the forest, mountain, or desert, to emphasize the healing by nature philosophy.

As the selected global Anglophone novels illustrate later in this book, the comparison between biomedicine and ethnomedicine does not express any preference, but argues in favor of their complementarity for a more competent healthcare. While biomedicine has achieved a revolutionary progress in the diagnosis and treatment of diseases and disabilities on empirical grounds, ethnomedicine has allowed an essential understanding of holistic healing practices that address the physical, emotional, sociocultural, and environmental dimensions of health and well-being. Integrating the culturally competent and ecologically oriented aspects of ethnomedicine into biomedicine offers a more comprehensive approach to healthcare that is centered on the care seeker.

There is, however, a growing tendency towards medical pluralism through the integration of biomedical and ethnomedical practices. Venera Khalikova names some new concept that are currently being used like medical "diversity," "syncretism," "hybridity," and "therapeutic itineraries," in which a care seeker chooses a personalized blend of biomedical and ethnomedical interventions. She says,

> In the context of today's globalisation, medical pluralism retains its analytical importance, especially in the examination of people's search for alternative cures locally and transnationally, the growing consumer market of 'holistic', 'traditional', and 'natural' treatments, and the attempts of many countries to incorporate alternative treatments into national healthcare. (1)

In this quote, the medical anthropologist shows the renewed interest in medical pluralism in the era of globalization and emphasizes the importance of Indigenous knowledge systems in alliance with the Euro-American-centric knowledge system.

The "doctor-patient" interaction can take various forms, based on factors such as communication styles, cultural considerations, and healthcare contexts. Thomas S. Szasz and Marc H. Hollender identify three models of "doctor-patient" relationships: "active-passivity" (parent-child), "guidance-co-operation" (parent-adolescent), and "mutual participation" (adult-adult). They explain the varying dynamics in this relationship that ranges from a paternalistic approach to a more collaborative and equal partnership; they call attention to the evolving nature of healthcare interactions that many healthcare providers around the world still overlook (586). The first two are doctor-centered and paternalistic models in which the healthcare recipient provides answers to medical questions and complies by prescribed treatments and instructions. The last model, however, highlights the benefits of a therapeutic alliance centered on the care seeker. Concerning culturally competent healthcare, as it occurs in ethnomedicine, there is an increasing belief that individuals from diverse cultural backgrounds have specific beliefs, values, and practices that affect their health and healthcare experiences. Significantly, the healthcare providers' "cultural competence" involves "understanding the importance of social and cultural influences on patients' health beliefs and behaviors" (Betancourt et al. 297). This competence allows them to offer respectful and effective care while also reducing healthcare disparities.

Regarding healthcare settings, a growing body of scientific research shows the importance of nature as it is illustrated in ethnomedicine. The historical roots of this idea are traced back to ancient Greece where nature was incorporated into healthcare settings. Contemporary Evidence-Based Design (EBD) relies on Roger S. Ulrich's article "View through a Window may Influence Recovery" (1984), in which he reports that individuals who have a view of greenery require reduced pain medication and experience shorter hospital stays when compared to those who have a view on brick walls (224). While many healthcare settings, especially in the Global South, cannot afford such idealistic conditions, they can create ambient environments through green colors, nature wall art, natural lights, and living plants.

A recent volume edited by Scott Slovic et al., *The Bloomsbury Handbook to Medical-Environmental Humanities* (2022), highlights "the power or symbiosis" that "lies with the hyphen," showing the "convergences, intersections–and [...] entanglements" between the medical and environmental humanities (6). In his "Introduction: Toward a Medical-Environmental Humanities: Why Now?" Slovic states that the emergence of the Covid-19 pandemic was clearly unwelcome as the authors were collaborating on their book. However, they realized the pressing need to integrate the two disciplines of medical humanities and environmental humanities (9). In their edited volume, they invite readers to reflect on the effects of increasingly hazardous climatic conditions on human health through the humanities. They shed light on environmental issues that directly affect human health and raise awareness about pollution, air and water quality, as well as their impacts on physical and mental well-being.

Intersectional studies conducted by ecofeminists show that women from marginalized communities, such as Indigenous or immigrant women, often face additional health risks due to environmental injustice. In Indigenous societies, women frequently handle household duties and take care of their family members' health. Vandana Shiva affirms, "women's involvement in the environmental movement has started with their lives and with the severe threat to the health of their families" (2). Ecofeminists thus seek to end these injustices, not only based on gender, but also on race and class. Arguing that the current environmental crisis is a result of patriarchal culture, Karen J. Warren perceives significant correlations between the subjugation of women and the subjugation of the environment; consequently, addressing ecological issues requires the incorporation of a feminist standpoint. She observes that mainstream masculine discourse often gives feminine attributes to nature and environmental attributes to women. "Mother Nature" and "Mother Earth," for instance, are usually depicted in feminine and even sexual terms, as she explains,

> Women are described in animal terms as pets, cows, sows, foxes, chicks, serpents, bitches, beavers, old bats, old hens, mother hens, pussycats, cats, cheetahs, bird-brains, and hare-brains…'Mother Nature' is raped, mastered, conquered, mined; her secrets are 'penetrated,' her 'womb' is to be put into the service of the 'man of science.' Virgin timber is felled, cut down; fertile soil is tilled, and land that lies 'fallow' is 'barren,' useless. The exploitation of nature and animals is justified by feminizing them; the exploitation of women is justified by naturalizing them. (27).

In this regard, ecofeminist and postcolonial feminists find a common ground in the rejection of established hierarchical and patriarchal systems dominated by the hegemonic white or colored male. They describe their situation as "double colonization," in which they are oppressed because of their gender, race, and class. They thus call attention to woman's ability for ecological conservation, owing to the existence of woman/nature symbolic connections.

Along the ecofeminist approach to health humanities, there is a growing feminist approach, in broader terms, to health humanities. Carla Tsampiras and Alex Müller, in their article "Overcoming 'Minimal Objectivity' and 'Inherent Bias': Ethics and Understandings of Feminist Research in a Health Sciences Faculty in South Africa" (2018), discuss the difficulties they encountered when attempting to teach a course on intersectional identities to medical students. The ethics committee justified the rejection by a lack of "minimal objectivity" and existence of an "inherent bias." The authors challenged the decision by creating room for "disciplinary curiosity" and "epistemic generosity" (1). This strategy aligns with feminist research approaches that frequently promote the subversion of established hierarchies and power systems in academia.

In "The Role of Feminist Health Humanities Scholarship and Black Women's Artistry in Re-Shaping the Origin Narrative of Modern, U.S. Gynecology" (2021), Rachel Dudley relies on black feminist studies to examine "the poetics and politics of remembering and forgetting – in relation to the origin narrative of modern U.S. gynecology." She relates James Marion Sims' experiments (1845–1849) on the three black slaves, Anarcha, Lucy, and Betsey, on whose unanesthetized bodies he developed the duckbill speculum and some surgical techniques. Notwithstanding the use of their bodies as an experimental terrain, he was recognized as "the father of modern gynecology." Dudley enumerates the humanities scholars, mainly black women artists, who have engaged in "the politics and poetics of counter-hegemonic storytelling" by considering the three slaves as "the mothers of modern gynecology," highlighting the particular role of poetry in "socio-medical meaning-making" (1–2). In 2019, following decades of protest, James Marion Sims' memorial in Central Park, New York City, was replaced by Vinnie Bagwell's sculpture "Victory beyond Sims," honoring the lives of Anarcha, Lucy, and Betsey.

Along similar lines of inclusivity in the field of global health humanities, there is an increasing interest in disability or crip studies[9] to tackle the lived experiences of people with disabilities in relation to health and healthcare. The 1980s saw the emergence of disability studies in the UK and the USA from the efforts of activists

---

9 Crip, short for cripple, has been used by disability activists to subvert the societal exclusion inherent in the word "disabled."

who analyzed the societal representations of disability. It studies "the social meanings, symbols, and stigmas attached to disability identity and asks how they relate to enforced systems of exclusion and oppression" (Siebers 3). While biomedicine adheres to a medical paradigm of disability that considers impairment as a person's physical dysfunction, disability studies undermines the prevalent models of disability and advances a more empowering perspective. It emphasizes the social model that views impairment as a result of physical, social, and cultural barriers affecting the person with the impairment. By criticizing ableism, the prevalent prejudice and discrimination towards people with disabilities, it draws attention to the connections between ableism and other types of discrimination based on race, gender, and class.

Conclusion

This is where, through the aforementioned inclusivity, an intersectional approach comes into health humanities. Because modern biomedicine is historically laden with issues of power, a global and inclusive approach "requires acknowledging that there are many ways of being and doing, unlearning the universality of being and actively engaging with pluriversalities of being" (Affun-Adegbulu and Adegbulu 3). To make it happen, global health humanities scholars and practitioners should acquire understanding on how race, gender, and class intersect to cause health inequalities. By comprehending the interconnections between different dimensions of human identity and valuing diverse backgrounds thanks to biomedicine, ethnomedicine, and health humanities, a more equitable global health can come true. Global health and global health humanities are increasingly addressing the relationship between biological, psychological, and social factors in the promotion of well-being and the achievement of equitable health outcomes.

2 Health Humanities and Global Anglophone Literature

Introduction

This book rests on the premise that the study of literature not only enhances clinical empathy and holistic care among healthcare students and professionals, but also promotes knowledge of existential themes like disease, disability, death, caregiving, health, and well-being among students and readers of literature. This is even more useful with an inclusive approach that gives voice to global Anglophone literature and shows the manner in which race, gender, and class intersect to cause inequalities in the field of health. For Italo Calvino, "the grand challenge of literature" in the third millennium "is to be capable of weaving together the various branches of knowledge, the various 'codes,' into a manifold and multifaceted vision of the world" (112). Calvino's words reflect a useful awareness of the role of literature in raising awareness about the world, emphasizing the need for it to evolve in interaction with the ever-expanding sources of knowledge. Literature has the potential of transcending disciplinary boundaries and offering a holistic perspective on the world, reflecting a multidimensional reality and fostering a deeper understanding of the interconnectedness of human existence. This chapter traces the long-standing alliance and narrative intersection between literature and medicine, highlighting the spirit of inclusivity in the field of global health humanities.

Literature and Medicine: A Time-honored Alliance

Literature has always sought to explore the nature of human existence, and medicine is an integral part of the web of life, involving the two disciplines in a perpetual dialogue. The fragility and impermanence of human life are common concerns in medicine. In a similar vein, existential questions related to the purpose of life and mortality of humans have long been intriguing themes in literature. In Greek mythology, Apollo, also called "Apollo Medicus" (Apollo the physician), was believed to possess the power to heal and protect from disease; he was worshipped as the supreme being of poetry and music, often portrayed playing a lyre. In the heyday of the Islamic civilization, scientists were polymaths like Ibn Sina (980–1037), known as Avicenna. The Persian polymath wrote *Al-Qanun fi'l-Tibb* (*The Canon of Medicine*), covering a wide range of medical topics intended as a comprehensive guide for medical education. His primary vocation was medicine, but he excelled in philosophy, mathematics, astronomy, and poetry. He developed a didactic approach to teaching medical knowledge through rhythmic verse to facilitate memorization, and he summarized his encyclopedic oeuvre into a 1326-verse poem, "*Al-Urjuzah Fi Al-Tibb*" (poem on medicine), which contributed to the transfer of his medical knowledge to Medieval Europe (Abdel-Halim 1).

In this discussion of the time-honored alliance between literature and medicine, it is important to highlight the role of physician-writers who create bridges between the two disciplines. By virtue of their medical vocation, they have access to the most private and vulnerable times in their care seekers' lives, sometimes at the brink of death. Using the writing vocation, they bear witness to existential situations that ordinary writers may never experience, and through fiction, they instruct readers on disease etiology, prevention, and treatment. In the Euro-American literary tradition, examples abound of physician-writers like John Keats, Arthur Conan Doyle, William Carlos Williams, Oliver Sacks, and William Somerset Maugham, to cite only a few. Their cases reflect the oft-quoted sentence by Anton Chekhov, in which he intimates, "medicine is my lawful, wedded wife, and literature is my mistress" (qtd. in McLellan 1618). In a metaphorical language, this passage highlights the author's relation with the two disciplines. The mention of marriage shows a sense of obligation and dedication to his medical profession while the reference to literature as his mistress gives it a position of passion and excitement in his life. While physician-writers draw on their practice of medicine when they write, countless non-physician writers also address the themes of disease and disability to examine their effects on both the individual and society.

Additionally, some care seekers write narratives, called pathographies, in which they relate their experiences. One of the most read books of this genre is Paul Kalanithi's *When Breath Becomes Air*, published posthumously in 2016. The caregiver turned care seeker explores the overpowering shift in perspective that occurs when a healthcare provider contracts an incurable disease. Kalanithi poignantly captures his journey from being an ingenious neurosurgeon who treated patients with life-threatening conditions to suddenly finding himself with terminal lung cancer at the age of 36. In eloquent prose, he reflects on the meaning of existence and the fragility of human life, and as he combats his own disease, he recalls the challenges, fears, and uncertainties that his care seekers used to face, showing his knowledge about disease from both sides of the equation. Such pathographies offer an intimate access to the experience of disease and disability, with their psychological and sociocultural implications that cannot be perceived in daily interactions. Readers get a glimpse of the lives of those who struggle with disease or disability, be it ever so authentic, and by vicariously experiencing their suffering, they develop much-needed empathy and tolerance. Readers hence project themselves onto the narratives, reflecting on their own lives, values, and priorities; this introspection is conducive to psychological resilience and empowerment.

Literature, with its unparalleled potential to weave narratives and evoke deep emotions, holds within its pages the power to probe into the meaning of human existence. In the field of medical ethics, which is filled with moral dilemmas, literature can serve as a masterful teacher, eliciting reflection and empathy. On the one hand, literature provides examples of altruistic and self-sacrificing physicians who can jeopardize their own lives to save other people. An example of these is Dr. Rieux in *The Plague* (1947) by Albert Camus; he is a dedicated physician who works selflessly during the outbreak of a plague in the Algerian city of Oran. On the other hand, literature provides examples of substandard physicians who serve as cautionary tales to explore issues in medical ethics like cupidity, carelessness, or abuse of power. An example of these is Dr. Henry Jekyll in *Dr. Jekyll and Mr. Hyde* (1886) by Robert Louis Stevenson; he concocts a potion that metamorphoses him by night into the monstrous Mr. Edward Hyde, showing the duality of man and the peril of unethical science.

Narrative Intersections of Literature and Medicine

Philosopher Alasdair MacIntyre, in his influential book *After Virtue: A Study in Moral Theory*, states, "man is in his actions and practice, as well as in his fictions, essentially a story-telling animal, [...] a teller of stories that aspire to truth." In his view, stories teach virtues because "there is no way to give us an understanding of any society, [...] except through the stock of stories which constitute its initial dramatic resources" (216). The view that human beings are storytelling creatures, *homo narrans*, has given birth to narrative psychology, which studies the "storied nature of human conduct." Theodore R. Sarbin first used this phrase in the title of his edited volume *Narrative Psychology: The Storied Nature of Human Conduct* (1986), in which the authors examine the value of storytelling in defining the self, giving meaning to life, recalling the past, making sense of the present, and envisioning the future.

Narrative has a healing potential that is reminiscent of Aristotle's "catharsis" and Sigmund Freud's "talking cure."[10] As stated by American philosopher Daniel

---

[10] "Catharsis," the Greek term for "purgation," refers to the "therapeutic effect" of tragedy upon spectators; "after the storm and climax there comes a sense of release from tension" (Cuddon 115). "Talking cure" refers to the process by which a care seeker articulates "the blockage of a pathogenic affect, resulting in its transportation from the 'inside' to the 'outside' and, eventually, a cathartic purgation" (Marx et al. 6).

Dennett, "no matter what atrocities are being narrated, the act of storytelling offers us an implicit narrative of survival to cling to, a post-trauma perspective with which to identify, and an absolute distinction between 'now' and 'then' which cordons off the narrated suffering" (418). This statement highlights the power of storytelling to provide solace in the face of atrocities. Regardless of the horrors being depicted, it offers a narrative of resilience and a lens through which an individual can identify with post-trauma perspectives, creating a lucid distinction between the present conditions and past afflictions being narrated.

As the study of selected novels later demonstrates, unhealed historical trauma haunts the characters until it is holistically treated: physically, mentally, emotionally, and spiritually. Psychoanalyst Viktor Frankl seems particularly relevant in this regard, especially with his concept of "logotherapy," a combination of the Greek words "logos" (which both means "the will of God" and "the word") and "therapeia" (healing). "Logotherapy" consequently refers to the process of healing through both faith and language. Frankl believes that human existence has three elements: the body, the mind, and the soul. Medicine and psychology treat the diseases of the body and the mind, but effective healing should equally include "the spiritual resources of the patient" (140). Aspects of Frankl's "logotherapy" include reconnections not only with relatives and friends, but more importantly, with nature and God. For instance, Native American ceremonial rites are "logotherapeutic" because they adopt an integrative approach to healing. They seek wholeness through physical, emotional, and spiritual balance, as well as through harmonious relationships with the family, community, and nature.

Global Anglophone literature usually serves a logotherapeutic role; it often reflects personal and social tragedies that seek recognition in the forms of testimonial narratives because literature has the ability to transmit the unspeakable suffering through figurative language. Suzette Henke, who considers the 20th century as "a century of historical trauma" (xi), shows the importance of "scriptotherapy," i.e., the process of writing the traumatic experience for a therapeutic purpose (xii). In her view, through "the artistic replication of a coherent subject-position, the life-writing project generates a healing narrative that temporarily restores the fragmented self to an empowered position of psychological agency." Autobiography, in particular, is a powerful form of "healing narrative" because it helps the author "fashion an enabling discourse of testimony and self-revelation" (xvi). The global Anglophone novels analyzed in this book are, principally, reflections of their authors' life stories, by which they try to ease their own suffering.

Significantly, narrative medicine is a flourishing practice that seeks to cure human beings by paying greater attention to their life stories. Interest in narrative has grown exponentially in the field of health, mainly through the work of physician Rita Charon who founded the Division of Narrative Medicine at Columbia University in the City of New York in 2000. The concept has been widely embraced as a multidisciplinary effort to promote the applications of narrative practices in medical education and clinical treatment. It has gained considerable momentum in the global efforts to educate healthcare providers on humane and reflective practice. Charon et al. note the five goals that are achievable through the inclusion of literature in medical instruction:

1) Literary accounts of illness can teach physicians concrete and powerful lessons about the lives of sick people; 2) great works of fiction about medicine enable physicians to recognize the power and implications of what they do; 3) through the study of narrative, the physician can better understand patients' stories of sickness and his or her own personal stake in medical practice; 4) literary study contributes to physicians' expertise in narrative ethics; and 5) literary theory offers new perspectives on the work and the genres of medicine. (599)

Each of these goals, the authors specify, can be achieved with particular literary texts whose deep characterization of the diseased person, the good or bad physician as well as the metaphorical richness of setting and dialogue, can imaginatively reflect real-life healthcare situations. In addition, literary works examine ethical dilemmas in medical experimentation, quality of life, ethics of caregiving, and end-of-life decisions, stimulating existentialist reflections among healthcare professionals.

Central to Charon's narrative medicine approach is the practice of "close reading" she borrows from literature; it entails a thorough examination of the text to elucidate its many levels of meaning. In "Close Reading: The Signature Method of Narrative Medicine," she argues that it "helps narrative medicine to achieve its goals of justice in healthcare, participatory practice, egalitarian learning, and deep relationships in practice" (157). It explores the language needs and choices made by the care seeker that go beyond cursory examination. Healthcare professionals can learn about hidden meanings, feelings, and experiences that may not be visible in medical records or diagnostic tests by carefully examining their narrative. Healthcare providers' effective use of narrative can help care seekers understand medical knowledge and promote shared decision-making, reducing fear, building trust, and fostering optimism. As healthcare providers share their experiences with one another through case presentations, publications, and conferences, narrative serves beyond clinical practice and extends to professional development.

Ethical Intersections of Literature and Medicine

There is a growing understanding in modern medicine that centering the healthcare approach on the care seeker is necessary to get a more comprehensive picture of the effect of disease and disability on the person's body, mind, soul, and life as a whole. Oliver Sacks, British neurologist who wrote bestseller "clinical tales," argues that Hippocrates established the case history, defined as the description of "the natural history of disease," but:

> Such histories [...] tell us nothing about the individual and his history; they convey nothing of the person, and the experience of the person, as he faces, and struggles to survive, his disease. There is no 'subject' in a narrow case history; modern case histories allude to the subject in a cursory phrase ('a trisomic albino female of 21'), which could as well apply to a rat as a human being. (*The Man who Mistook* ix-x)

This passage emphasizes the critical limitation in Hippocrates' traditional case history that overlooks the care seeker's subjective experience. While it records the evidence-based features of the disease, the pathology, the case history dismisses its impacts on the mind and soul, somehow reducing humans to bodies or pathologies. Believing that literature can humanize these case histories by putting names, faces, and emotions on them, Sacks wrote "clinical tales" on patients suffering from various neurological disorders like migraine, encephalitis, Parkinson's disease, Tourette's syndrome, color blindness, etc. He writes, in a letter to Russian physician-writer Alexander Luria, "the vision of such a poetic science, a total fusion of Art and Science, grips my heart and my mind with equal force, and tantalizes with glimpses of an old unity restored" (Archives). Holding fast to Romantic medicine, he has been criticized as a scientific popularizer whose tales are a literary form of pseudo-science, but he insists that they provide a complementary perspective to standard neurology, not an alternative to it, springing from the human innate inclination for narrative.

Literature is, furthermore, important in the study of ethics cases, which are concise scenarios that raise moral dilemmas related to medical practice, including objective information about the patients, ethical quandaries, legal considerations, and clinical decisions. The medical student must determine what the healthcare provider ought to do, or not do; the goal is to stimulate reflection about potential ethical dilemmas before they actually happen in a high-stress clinical setting. In "Showing that Medical Ethics Cases Can Miss the Point," Woods Nash analyzes ethics cases that are common assignments for medical and nursing students. He argues that the conciseness of the ethics case often leads to a focus on action, sidelining the importance of character, context, and interaction. It is reductive because it does not account for the gray areas that often permeate real-life medical situations. Nash observes, "By comparing short story and case, we are led to wonder anew whether ethics cases that represent real events might also fail to probe to the heart of the matter. Thus, rewriting short stories as ethics cases can inculcate a healthy skepticism as to whether any case has succeeded in conveying what is most at stake" (190). He suggests that the act of rewriting short stories with ethical dilemmas can broaden the students' perspectives and make them more sensitive to the situation they might encounter in real life.

Since there is barely no reference to the subjectivity of the patient in the standard ethics case, the use of storytelling provides more room for contextualization. Fiction hence turns into what Frank Hakemulder considers as a moral laboratory in which "plausible implications of human conduct can be studied in a relatively controlled and safe way" (150). The experience of fictionality would free the medical student or practitioner from the usual state of cautious skepticism, which often serves as a barrier in real-life interactions. Marco Caracciolo hypothesizes that fictionality prompts readers to drop their defenses, thereby enhancing their ability to empathize with characters more readily than with real humans. This abstract divide between reality and fiction can serve as a protective space, encouraging readers to embrace experiential viewpoints that they would be less inclined to adopt in genuine interpersonal encounters (29). In this way, literature provides an immersive space that allows individuals to experiment with their moral sensibilities, explore ethical dilemmas, empathize with different perspectives, and challenge preconceived notions.

Health and Well-being in Global Anglophone Literature

Global Anglophone Literature is increasingly becoming a powerful instrument for addressing pressing concerns across the world, notably the enduring repercussions of slavery, colonialism, and migration. By extension, it can play an important role in the field of health humanities by exploring the historical, political, and sociocultural aspects of health and healthcare. By illustrating the distress of people with disease and disability in disadvantaged locations, with related healthcare disparities, it can reveal the flaws of healthcare systems and ignite discussions about global health equity.

The exploration of "corporeality" holds significance in the discussion of health and well-being in global Anglophone literature. It is better understood in this context if morphologically divided as "corpo-reality" rather than "corporeal-ity" to highlight the lived experience of the body in postcolonial societies. In their introduction to "The Body and Performance," Bill Ashcroft et al. compare the body to a text on which "colonisation has written some of its most graphic and scrutable messages" (322). The body, being a predominant feature of the colonial condition, stands "metonymically for all the 'visible' signs of difference, and their varied forms of cultural and social inscription" (321). To elucidate the enduring impact of colonialism on individuals, the authors employ the metaphor of the body as a palimpsest, a manuscript that has been overwritten, often with the original text partially or completely erased. They present the body as a metonym for all the visible signs of difference imposed by colonial powers.

Elleke Boehmer reinforces the statement that in colonial representation, exclusion is often visually represented through the colonized body. She writes:

> The seductive and repulsive qualities of the wild or other, as well as its punishment and expulsion from the community, are figured on the body, and as (fleshly, corporeal, often speechless) body. To rehearse some of the well-known binary tropes of postcolonial discourse, as opposed to the coloniser (white man, centre of intellection, of control), the other is cast as carnal, untamed, instinctual, raw, and therefore also open to mastery, available for use, for husbandry, for numbering, branding, cataloguing, possession, penetration. (129)

The body is, therefore, a space on which the experiences of colonization are inscribed and made visible. The silenced body refers to the suppression of the voice and agency of the colonized, and the wounded body refers to the physical and emotional toll inflicted upon them through forced labor, cruel torture, and lasting scars. Boehmer adds that the imagery associated with the body of the "other" is often intertwined with the imagery associated with unexplored land, depicted as wild, alluring, mysterious, and available for possession.

A recurrent corporeal metaphor in global Anglophone literature is the virus that alludes to the influence of outside forces that infect and corrupt native cultures. The metaphor of the monster is another one that stands in for the lasting effects of colonialism, still haunting independent countries or ethnic minorities in the form of abject poverty, social inequality, and political unrest. Another prevailing metaphor is the wound, which stands for the persistent traumatic stress that accompanies slavery, colonialism, or migration, as well as the ongoing struggles with regard to social injustice, rampant corruption, and political instability.

Trauma, which derives from the Greek word "titrosko"[11], refers to the psychic wound of an individual who suffered from tragic circumstances. According to Cathy Caruth, trauma includes "the symptoms of what had previously been called shell shock, combat stress, delayed stress syndrome, and traumatic neurosis," as a

---

[11] Trauma is the equivalent of the Greek word "tô rpaùpa" that is a "bodily injury or wound"; it is the noun form of the verb "titrosko" (TtTpœoKco) that means "to pierce, to wound" ("Etymological explorations").

response "to both human and natural catastrophes" (3). In the context of World War I and its aftermath, psychiatrists called it "battle fatigue" or "shell shock," but since World War II and the Vietnam War, they have called it "Post-Traumatic Stress Disorder" (PTSD) or Continuous Traumatic Stress Disorder (CTSD). It is defined as a "severe psychological disturbance following a traumatic event, characterised by the involuntary re-experiencing of the event combined with symptoms of hyperarousal, dissociation, and avoidance" (Geddes et al. 269). It includes, among others, post-traumatic slave syndrome, child abuse syndrome, rape trauma syndrome, battered women's syndrome, and it refers to the hallucinations, nightmares, and other symptoms that repeatedly bring up the traumatic event.

In this book, part of the interest lies in postcolonial trauma studies that emerged from the criticism directed against seminal trauma theories for being Eurocentric. Stef Craps believes that if the field has "any hope of redeeming its promise of ethical effectiveness," it has to be inclusive of subordinate groups ("Wor(l)ds" 53). He initiates the field of postcolonial trauma studies to explore the long-term psychological and sociocultural effects of colonialism on native populations. Drawing on Fanon's writing to advance a complementary approach that permits "visions of cross-cultural solidarity and justice" (*Postcolonial* 101), he believes that, in order to achieve its ethical aspiration, trauma studies must be urgently decolonized to take into account the different manifestations of traumatic suffering and their representations in literature.

Dissecting the "corporeal malediction" inflicted on the colonized by the colonizer in *Black Skin, White Masks*, Fanon uses the metaphor of amputation to bewail his own traumatic experience, "What else could it be for me but an amputation, an excision, a hemorrhage that spattered my whole body with black blood?" (112). He tells of "being dissected under white eyes," by the "galaxy of erosive stereotypes" (129) of those who "cut away slices of [his] reality" (116). He recounts how he felt his corporeality disintegrate after being objectified as "evil" in the gaze of a white child who screamed, "Mama, look at the Negro! I'm frightened!" (112). Fanon explains that the child's gaze "abraded" his body "into nonbeing" (109); that he "felt knife blades" open within him (118), and that his body was returned to him "sprawled out, distorted, recolored, clad in mourning" (113). The author uses powerful imagery to convey the dehumanizing and objectifying effects of the white gaze on the colored body. He compares the shock of encountering racial prejudice to polypsychism (psychic multiplication). He suggests that the colonized struggles with conflicting desires to maintain their original identity while also seeking approval from the colonizer. This internal struggle manifests as a tripartite conflict involving the self, the other, and a hybrid identity emerging from the collision of the two.

Metaphoric Representations of the Diseased Body

Metaphors are powerful literary tools used to represent the many-sided experiences of disease. They have a healing potential that lies in their capacity to transcend logic, to help human beings "perceive subtle and unusual connections, show relationships between outer experience and inner feeling, enable a sense of psychological and spiritual balance, open communication between known and unknown parts of [their] lives" (Burns and McKane 303). Metaphors help human beings describe elements of their lives that may be challenging to convey in literal terms; in other words, they are potent tools that enable them to make associations beyond the literal meaning and make sense of deep-seated emotions. In medicine and psychology, for instance, it is common among victims of Post-Traumatic Stress Disorder to use metaphors to express their traumatic experiences since they provide alternative frames of reference that help victims recall painful events without much suffering. Because trauma creates an inner conflict that resists direct representation, literature, with its figurative language, can voice the horror of traumatic experiences.

Susan Sontag, analyzing the use of illness metaphors in a variety of disciplines, including psychology, medicine, and literature, criticizes the manner that care seekers are surrounded by metaphorically discriminatory walls based on the ideology of health promotion. She writes, "My point is that illness is not a metaphor, and that the most truthful way of regarding illness – and the healthiest way of being ill – is one most purified of, most resistant to, metaphoric thinking" (*Illness* 3). The author condemns the tabooing of illness through metaphors and calls for the sterilization of discourse from their use because they foster exclusion and prejudice. For instance, she says, "illustrating the classic script for plague, AIDS is thought to have started in the 'dark continent,' then spread to Haiti, then to the United States and to Europe." It is viewed, as in colonial times, like "another infestation from the so-called Third World, which is after all where most people in the world live" (*AIDS* 51–52). Through such metaphors, the consideration that Africa is the cradle of AIDS fosters anti-African sentiments throughout the world and nurtures stereotypes about their sexual licentiousness. This is comparable to the "Yellow Peril" stereotype during the Covid-19 pandemic when anti-Asian sentiments resurfaced, blaming them for the health crisis because they ingest wild animals.

In light of this, it is important to show the semantic difference between disease, illness, and sickness, three "modes of unhealthy," according to Marshall Marinker, that are often used interchangeably while they carry some nuances. Disease is, for him, "a pathological process, most often physical as in throat infection, or cancer of the bronchus, sometimes undetermined in origin, as in schizophrenia. The quality which identifies disease is some deviation from a biological norm.

There is an objectivity about disease which doctors are able to see, touch, measure, smell." Illness, however, "is a feeling, an experience of unhealth which is entirely personal, interior to the person of the patient. Often it accompanies disease, but the disease may be undeclared, as in the early stages of cancer or tuberculosis or diabetes. Sometimes illness exists where no disease can be found." Sickness, ultimately, "is the external and public mode of unhealth. Sickness is a social role, a status, a negotiated position in the world, a bargain struck between the person henceforward called 'sick', and a society which is prepared to recognise and sustain him" (82–83). In these definitions, disease is a tangible manifestation that can be identified through medical examinations, illness is a subjective experience that is interior to the care seeker while sickness is a social perception and response to it. This semantic distinction highlights the importance of understanding the objective manifestations of diseases, the subjective experiences of illness, and the social dynamics of sickness to get the full picture of the medical condition.

Metaphoric Representations of the Disabled Body

Different disability models present divergent viewpoints on the nature and cause of disability, as well as the social perception of it. The medical model sees disability as an individual issue arising from the person's impairment, and in order to lessen the effects of this impairment on body functioning, it focuses on "repairing" it through medical interventions like chemical drugs, surgical operations, or other evidence-based therapies. Paul Hunt's *Stigma: The Experience of Disability* (1966) is a landmark in the field; he affirms in it that "The problem of disability lies not only in the impairment of function and its effects on us individually, but also, more importantly, in the area of our relationship with 'normal people' " (146). In this statement, the problem with disability extends beyond the physical limitations imposed on body functioning and points to the disabling interactions with those who are considered "normal." Hence comes the social model that views disability as an outcome of the interactions between people with impairments and discriminatory social conditions.

The Union of the Physically Impaired against Segregation (UPIAS) provides the following distinction between the concepts of "impairment" and "disability":

> [...] we define impairment as lacking part of or all of a limb, or having a defective limb, organ or mechanism of the body; and disability as the disadvantage or restriction of activity caused by a contemporary social organisation which takes no or little account of people who have physical impairments and thus excludes them from participation in the mainstream of social activities. Physical disability is therefore a particular form of social oppression. (20)

This distinction focuses on the social constraints that limit the full inclusion of people with disabilities and seeks to dismantle them to advance accessibility, inclusivity, and equality. The biopsychosocial model, explained in Chapter One, bridges the medical and social models by integrating the biological, psychological, and social components that affect disability (Hogan E16). It admits that psychological and social factors exacerbate the individual's bodily dysfunction, and it emphasizes the need for a holistic approach to treatment.

Disability studies garnered acclaim as a distinct academic discipline in the 1980s. Since then, academics have analyzed the perceptions of the "ab/normal" body in literature, examining works on disability and its metaphorical representations. Literary disability studies emerged in this activist climate to shed light on the common stereotypes conveyed by literary works to debunk their fallacious arguments. In their seminal book, *Narrative Prosthesis: Disability and the Dependencies of Discourse* (2000), David T. Mitchell and Sharon L. Snyder argue that disability serves as "the master trope of human disqualification" (3) because it stands for "a panoply of other social maladies that writers seek to address" (17). Supporting their arguments by examples from Herman Melville's *Moby Dick* (1851), Katherine Dunn's *Geek Love* (1989) and others, they decry the employment of disability as an "opportunistic metaphorical device" (47), as a "crutch upon which literary narratives lean for the representational power, disruptive potentiality, and analytical insight" (49). Mitchell and Snyder use the concept of "narrative prosthesis" as a theoretical framework to investigate the function of disability as a "prosthetic" plot device, complementing the narrative of able-bodied characters, maintaining ableist attitudes towards people with disabilities, and portraying them as objects of pity instead of fully realized individuals. By leaning on disability as a metaphorical "crutch," therefore, some literary narratives gain the ability to symbolically represent various societal issues.

Reinforcing the arguments of Mitchell and Snyder, Stuart Murray writes, "Stereotypical narrative scripts have the potential to reinforce ableist conceptions of disability as an absence; disabled characters are [...] often used merely as a tool to reveal something about the non-disabled protagonists" (249). This quotation emphasizes a critical assessment of stereotyped narratives that normalize ableism by treating disability as a flaw. Frequently, characters with disabilities serve only as plot devices to make other characters appear more compelling, ignoring their own deep and varied experiences. Lennard Davis contends that this notion of disability as just an instrument to reinforce the norm is valid not only at the character level but also at the genre level; he argues that the novel is a fundamentally normative genre that can influence people's conceptions of disability. He explains:

[...] the very structures on which the novel rests tend to be normative, ideologically emphasizing the universal quality of the central character whose normativity encourages us to identify with him or her. Furthermore, the novel's goal is to reproduce, on some level, the semiologically normative signs surrounding the reader, that paradoxically help the reader to read those signs in the world as well as the text. The middleness of life, the middleness of the material world, the middleness of the normal body, the middleness of a sexually gendered, ethnically middle world is created in symbolic form and then reproduced symbolically. ("Constructing Normalcy" 11)

For Davis, therefore, the novel is one of the "public venues" where the "abnormal" is useful to foster domination in relation to disability, race, gender, and class, thereby constructing normalcy of the white, upper-class, and able-bodied male. Leonard Kriegel also observes that literature has historically presented disability as a source of compassion or menace, with little to be added to the two stereotypes (31). Yet, despite the certainty that literary works have used such binary representations of disability, claiming that these are the only two attitudes involves an oversimplification.

Ato Quayson's *Aesthetic Nervousness: Disability and the Crisis of Representation* (2007), one of the most important books in literary disability studies, deals with the representations of disability in African American, Irish, Nigerian, and South African literature. What he calls "aesthetic nervousness" happens "when the dominant protocols of representation within the literary text are short-circuited in relation to disability" (15). In the primary level, it lies in the interactions and tensions between characters with disabilities and other characters. In a secondary level, it is increased by the use of symbols and motifs, as well as narrative devices or dramatic techniques. Aesthetic nervousness can also lie in the relationship between the text and the reader who witnesses the trials and tribulations of a character with a disability against the backdrop of social preconceptions (15). As opposed to Kriegel's reductionist classification of disability, limited to two options, Quayson creates a typology of nine representations, with countless intersections in between (table 2):

Table 2: Ato Quayson's Typology of Disability Representation

Type	Description
1 "*Disability as null set and/or moral test*" (37)	The character with a disability serves as a kind of moral foreground to the other characters, or as a way to measure or improve their moral standing. For example, Circe in Toni Morrison's *Song of Solomon* is a powerful wheelchair user who, through wisdom and

Table 2: Ato Quayson's Typology of Disability Representation *(Continued)*

Type	Description
	healing abilities, serves as a catalyst for the self-discovery and transformation of the protagonist.
2 *"Disability as the interface with otherness (race, class, sexuality, and social identity)"* (39)	In this type, the character with a disability is a signifier of a stark otherness and moral deficit; in their meeting, the protagonist reaches self-discovery of a superior status. For example, in Robert Louis Stevenson's *Treasure Island*, Blind Pew and Long John Silver the pirates are characters with disabilities who serve as foils to Jim Hawkins, the heroic, able-bodied main character.
3 *"Disability as articulation of disjuncture between thematic and narrative vectors"* (41)	In this type, the disconnection between content and form revolves around the character with a disability. For instance, in Bapsi Sidhwa's *Cracking India*, Lenny acts like an adult when she addresses the reader, but she remains a child in her interactions with the other characters of the novel, a contradiction that, for Quayson, verges on the implausible.
4 *"Disability as bearer of moral deficit/evil"* (42)	In this type, the character with a disability is described as a villain. In William Shakespeare's *The Tempest*, for instance, Caliban is a misshapen slave whose disability represents otherness as moral deficit.
5 *"Disability as epiphany"* (45)	In this type, sudden revelation and special knowledge emanate from disability. For example, in Harper Lee's *To Kill a Mockingbird*, Tom Robinson's disability is not revealed to the reader until the pivotal court scene where he is unjustly accused of raping a white girl. The narrative reveals that he could not have choked Mayella and caused the handprint bruises on her neck because of his crippled arm.
6 *"Disability as signifier of ritual insight"* (47)	This type has a ritual dimension; it views disability as a vehicle of spiritual insight, and the character with a disability as possessing a special bond with the divine. Society needs the benefit that such characters possess, deemed essential for its well-being. For instance, Wole Soyinka's plays feature Eshu, the hobbling trickster deity of the crossroads in Yoruba culture; his limp serves as a metaphor for access to both the material world and the world of the deities.

Table 2: Ato Quayson's Typology of Disability Representation *(Continued)*

Type	Description
7 *"Disability as inarticulable and enigmatic tragic insight"* (49)	In this type, disability resists understanding, and the character with a disability is usually depicted as having a tragic feature that is not easy to verbalize. Most frequently, this character is a female, as Consolata in Toni Morrison's *Paradise*. Besides the race and class perspectives in literary works of this type, gender produces a dialectical coupling of sorrowful insight and voice deprivation.
8 *"Disability as hermeneutical impasse"* (50)	In this type, disability resists interpretation, challenging readers' assumptions and urging them to struggle with the equivocation of disability. For instance, in Michael Ondaatje's *The English Patient*, David Caravaggio, maimed during WWII and under morphine addiction, is desperately looking for the truth, and he cannot even remember his own name.
9 *"Disability as normality"* (52)	In this type, the character with a disability is a normal human being, with the full gamut of emotions, paradoxes, desires, and anxieties. For instance, in *The Body Silent*, Robert Murphy chronicles his subjective views of his disability as well as the social reactions to it, and despite signs of aesthetic nervousness in the text, the emphasis remains on the social critique rather than the disability itself.

An important book in the field of postcolonial disability studies is *Postcolonial Fiction and Disability: Exceptional Children, Metaphor and Materiality* (2011), in which Clare Barker calls for more attention to literature outside of the Euro-American canon to discover other cultural perspectives on disability. She uses Mitchell and Snyder's concept of "narrative prosthesis" to explain the use of disability as a metaphor in five postcolonial novels: Patricia Grace's *Potiki*, Tsitsi Dangarembga's *Nervous Conditions* and *The Book of Not*, Bapsi Sidhwa's *Cracking India*, Salman Rushdie's *Midnight Children*, and Ben Okri's *The Famished Road*. She argues that this approach informs her readings because it reveals "the relationship between metaphor and materiality that is so crucial to the 'disabled child-nation' phenomenon, and providing an appropriately politicized theoretical framework from which to approach it" (19). The narrators of the five novels are children with disabilities, symbolizing that colonialism is responsible for important damage in the young nations. Regardless of the disability that characterizes the five children, this child-nation metaphor is quite demeaning for the newly independent countries. However, Barker shows that these children with disabilities possess qualities that challenge normative narratives; they have potential for psychological growth and societal transformation.

The previous examples highlight the duality of literature and its impact on the sociocultural perceptions of disability. On the one hand, it can reinforce societal norms and stereotypes surrounding disability, perpetuating the status quo of what is considered "normal." On the other hand, literature also serves as a powerful tool of resistance by challenging the established perceptions of disability and offering alternative narratives. In Alice Hall's words, it "has the potential to reach large and diverse populations; it serves a pedagogic function in the sense that it not only documents but also shapes attitudes towards disability" (4). It can urge readers to question traditional perceptions of normalcy and disability by featuring empowered characters with disabilities, thus nurturing empathy and ensuring inclusivity of the full spectrum of human experiences.

In "Disability Haunting in American Poetics," Snyder and Mitchell highlight the potential of literature in providing imaginative "intimacy" with characters who suffer from disabilities against the backdrop of their social marginalization (6). The imaginary exposure with such characters can create an empathetic connection and clear understanding of their conditions in real-life situations, especially if they face other types of societal exclusion based on race, gender, or class. In *Extraordinary Bodies: Figuring Physical Disability in American Literature and Culture*, Rosemarie Garland-Thomson celebrates African American women's "liberatory" novels about disability written by Toni Morrison and Audre Lorde (6). With their strong and resilient characters, they deconstruct the stereotype that having a disability reduces one's agency and attractiveness. For instance, in Morrison's *Sula*, a poor African American female amputee, named Eva Peace, has a charismatic personality that defies societal expectations. Through her example, Morrison provides a counter-narrative that celebrates the potential of persons with disabilities living in marginalized groups.

Leading literary disability studies scholars argue that the largest obstacle the field is currently facing is the necessity to move from universalism to cultural diversity. Snyder and Mitchell contend that it needs to:

> [...] grow more international in its critique (and less Eurocentric in its models). The future of the field depends upon its ability to take up this challenge in a way that does not replicate the global commodification of other identities. This entails a thoroughgoing recognition that Western-based methodologies have limited utility for apprehending disability in other cultural contexts. (*Cultural Locations* 198–199)

Even if "Western" perspectives have made a substantial contribution to the field, the authors believe, it is important to recognize their shortcomings and the value of embracing "non-Western" viewpoints and Indigenous knowledge systems. This inclusive method provides a heightened understanding of disability that takes into account the various historical and sociocultural settings in which it exists.

The postcolonial theory offers an alternative lens through which disability can be understood, providing an inclusive perspective that challenges the master narratives. Postcolonial and disability studies have a common concern for the "silenced populations" (Hunt 47); both of them place a strong emphasis on the experiences of oppressed and underprivileged individuals whose voices are suppressed within the dominant discourse. Postcolonial studies looks at the effects of colonialism and imperialism as well as the power dynamics between the dominant and the dominated, aiming to undermine the prevailing master narratives that have nurtured the imbalance of power. Disability studies also denounces the effects of stereotypes and highlights the perspectives of people with disabilities with a view to dismantling ableist systems. Both postcolonial studies and disability studies aspire to deconstruct the power structures that keep their target populations on the margins in order to promote social justice and inclusion.

As a result, the goal of postcolonial disability studies is to comprehend the experiences of people with disabilities not only in the Global South, but also in Indigenous communities and other ethnic minorities in the Global North. As it happens, it is estimated that 400 million of people with disabilities, between 66 and 75 percent of the world's number of persons with disabilities, live in the Global South (Goodley 39). Helen Meekosha explains the "multiplicity of phenomena" that led to these numbers, comprising "war and civil strife, nuclear testing, the growth of the arms trade, the export of pollution to 'pollution havens' and the emergence of sweatshops" (667). These factors highlight the sociopolitical and economic dynamics that influence the frequency of disabilities in the Global South. For instance, wars result in numerous injuries and poor access to healthcare, hence increasing the number of disabilities. The use of weapons results in bodily damage while nuclear testing and pollution expose people to dangerous substances that cause impairments and chronic health problems. Sweatshops, usually industries from the Global North delocalized in the Global South, are known for exploitative labor practices that cause occupational hazards. The previous examples connect the various dimensions of environmental imperialism, shedding light on how global power dynamics influence the health and abilities of populations in the Global South.

Conclusion

Literature has the power to transcend barriers and touch readers from diverse backgrounds and perspectives. It can shape attitudes towards people with disease and disability by offering alternative narratives, highlighting their resilience, and providing the possibility for their stories to be shared. By portraying them in authentic ways, it can dismantle stereotypes and promote tolerance and empathy among readers. Adopting the global health humanities approach to the study of the global Anglophone novel offers a challenging perspective on the effects of the colonial encounter on medical knowledge, as well as the power dynamics between the colonizers and the colonized in relation to healthcare. This approach also provides a better understanding of cultural differences in the conception of disease, disability, health, and well-being. In so doing, literature can ideally influence public opinion and shape political decisions, contributing to the promotion of a more inclusive and equitable global health.

Part II: Infectious Diseases in the Global Anglophone Novel

1 Virgin Soil Epidemics and Unresolved Traumatic Grief in Louise Erdrich's *Tracks*

Introduction

Louise Erdrich's *Tracks* (1988) traces the grave history of the Anishinabe community from 1912 to 1924 in North Dakota, through deadly epidemics of influenza, smallpox, and tuberculosis, with associated trauma and starvation. It illustrates the inspirational Dakota proverb, "We will be forever known by the tracks we leave," and suggests that virgin soil epidemics, unresolved grief, and Indigenous healing traditions will continue to shape the cultural identity and collective memory of Native Americans. By weaving stories of survivance, Erdrich skillfully subverts the prevailing narratives that glorify imperial expansion as Manifest Destiny.

Virgin Soil Epidemics

When Christopher Columbus arrived in what is now called the Americas in 1492, he encountered a vast land and a diverse population grouped into over five hundred tribes that had been living there for centuries. Their sociocultural structures, characterized by hunting and gathering for sustenance, were deeply grounded in the environment; the arrival of European settlers changed their lives and the lands they called home. The first settlers could not survive the first winters without the help of the Natives who provided shelter, food, and remedies. The encounter, however, was woeful for the Native American populations; it is estimated that 80–95 percent were wiped out in the 100–150 years after 1492 (Nunn and Qian 165).

This encounter caused what historians commonly call the "Columbian Exchange," referring to the bartering of goods, plants, animals, and diseases, between Europe and America in the early times of settlement. Regarding diseases, the first aspect of the exchange is probably the transmission of syphilis from Caribbean populations to Europeans, but the transmission was more destructive in the opposite direction. Indigenous populations were vulnerable to the introduction of new viruses and diseases transported from Europe because they had been isolated from the rest of the world for thousands of years. This is known as the "virgin soil epidemics" defined by Alfred W. Crosby as those with which "the populations at risk have had no previous contact," and to which they were "immunologically almost defenseless," adding that "a number of dangerous maladies – smallpox, measles, malaria, yellow fever, and undoubtedly several more – were unknown in the pre-Columbian New World ("Virgin" 289). In *Ecological Imperialism: The Biological Expansion of Europe*, Crosby further explains the impact of European diseases as a bio-geographical factor on the success of colonialism, meaning that the pathogens played a primary role in displacing Indigenous populations and enabling the demographic dominance of "Neo-Europe" (196).

Medical research archives document a consistent pattern of epidemic outbreaks among Indigenous American tribes spanning centuries. The records highlight their vulnerability to epidemics that were not associated with one pathogen spreading over less than a decade. Rather, different pathogens led to successive waves of virgin soil epidemics insofar as individuals who survived one epidemic, such as influenza, would later die from another, such as smallpox. Those who survived both could potentially be affected by subsequent waves of diseases like measles (Koch et al. 22–24). The 16th-century illustration below (figure 5) shows Indigenous Americans infected by the smallpox virus and "wrapped in blankets, they are covered with pustules, their agony registered in their faces and body positions. One patient is crying out in pain, while another is receiving consolation from a woman" (Fields 14). This illustration captures the Indigenous peoples' suffering and agony, as well as their compassionate act of mutual consolation.

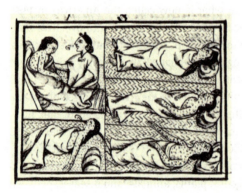

Figure 5: Nahuas Infected with Smallpox (16th century) (Public domain image from *Florentine Codex*, reproduced from Fields 14)

Knowing about the vulnerability of Indigenous tribes to viruses, Jeffery Amherst, leader of British forces during the French and Indian War (1754–1763), allegedly waged "germ warfare" against them by distributing smallpox-infected blankets. During Pontiac's War (1763), the general commanded, "You will do well to try to inoculate the Indians by means of blankets, as well as to try every other method that can serve to extirpate this execrable race." William Trent, trader and officer, noted in his journal during the Siege of Fort Pitt in the same year, "Out of our regard to them we gave them two blankets and a handkerchief out of the Small Pox Hospital. I hope it will have the desired effect" (qtd. in Ranlet 428). These two quotes, with their disturbing contemptuous tone, are a testament on the history of imperialism in which diseases were weaponized to eradicate indigenous populations. The expansionist agenda was therefore tarnished by irreparable damage inflicted upon Indigenous tribes in the name of Manifest Destiny (see figure 6), a concept that emerged in the 19th century to assert the divine mission of the United States to expand its territorial boundaries from coast to coast.

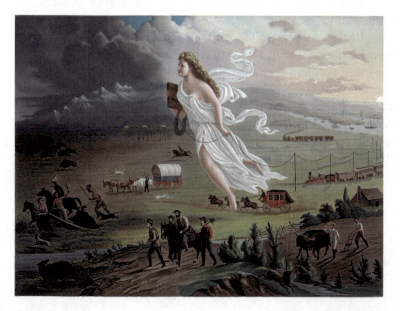

Figure 6: John Gast's "American Progress" as an Allegory of Manifest Destiny (Public domain illustration in Geo. A. Crofutt's *Trans-Continental Tourist*. picturinghistory.gc.cuny.edu/john-gast-american-progress-1872/)

Erdrich's *Tracks* is an illustration of Native Americans' need to "tell their stories and their own histories" (Peterson 985) from their perspective as victims. The novel commences by depicting the relentless onslaught of smallpox and tuberculosis epidemics that ravaged Anishinabe tribes. The first chapter unfolds through the narrative voice of Nanapush, the medicine man, and portrays his tribe's arduous journey towards recovery. He recounts, "We started dying before the snow, and like the snow, we continued to fall. It was surprising there were so many of us left to die. [...] that disease must have claimed all of the Anishinabe that the earth could hold and bury" (Erdrich 1). The passage refers to the smallpox outbreak of 1912 that resulted in a considerable loss of lives. Despite the severity of the epidemic, there were individuals who miraculously managed to survive. Unfortunately, the challenges persisted beyond that, as a subsequent epidemic of "consumption" (tuberculosis) emerged, further exacerbating the hardships faced by the population. Nanapush carries on, "A new sickness swept down. The consumption. [...] whole families of your relatives lay ill and helpless in its breath. On the reservation, where we were forced close together, the clans dwindled. [...] My own family was wiped out one by one" (2). This poignant passage eloquently illustrates the recurrence of diverse infectious diseases in the backdrop of broken treaties and land removal, resulting in the near annihilation of the Native American community.

In *Tracks*, Nanapush embodies the spirit of *midewiwin* (see figure 7), translated as the Grand Medicine Society, a spiritual group in the Anishinaabe tribes of the Upper Great Lakes, northern prairies, and eastern subarctic regions (Powell 159). For their ancestral wisdom, *midew* healers act as intermediaries between the human and spirit worlds, as well as between community members in governance, decision-making, and conflict resolution. While this tradition has almost been exterminated by colonial settlement and forced assimilation, it has managed to survive, and there are presently active *midewiwin* doom-roofed lodges where medicine men cure the Anishinaabe community.

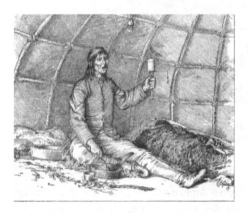

Figure 7: Ojibwe *Midew* (Medicine Man) in a *Mide-wiigiwaam* (Medicine Lodge) (Public domain image, reproduced from Powell 159)

Nanapush preserves the healing traditions of his tribe by skillfully diagnosing illnesses and employing the power of meaningful chants and stories to bring healing to those going through bereavement. When "the consumption" spreads among the community, he calls it "the invisible sickness" and traces its origin to *windigo*, the evil spirit in Anishinaabe mythology. He might be referring to the white man as living with *wetiko* psychosis, a disease of cannibalism, whose symptoms include vanity, cupidity, enslavement, genocide, and relentless exploitation of the planet's resources. Native American historian Jack D. Forbes, in his controversial book titled *Columbus and Other Cannibals: The Wetiko Disease of Exploitation, Imperialism and Terrorism*, writes, "*Wétiko* is a Cree term (*windigo* in Ojibway, *wintiko* in Powhatan) which refers to a cannibal or, more specifically, to an evil person or spirit who terrorizes other creatures by means of terrible evil acts, including cannibalism" (24). Nanapush, in this perspective, challenges the prevailing notion of the "Savage Indian" by turning the tables and applying the term "*windigo*/cannibal" to the Euro-American settlers who transmitted the destructive diseases.

Like Nanapush, Fleur is a medicine woman whose whole family perished "in the last scourge of sickness" (Erdrich 6); she has inherited "the secret ways to cure or kill" (2) and committed to preserve the "half-forgotten medicines" (12). She has, as a resilient Native American woman, an overwhelming strength during her labor provoked by the intrusion of a bear; she elevates herself on a stack of blankets and brings forth the child. A woman "packed wormwood and moss between her legs, wrapped her in blankets heated with stones, then kneaded Fleur's stomach and forced her to drink cup after cup of boiled raspberry leaf" (60). The new mother releases a deep groan and cradles her daughter, Lulu, to her breast. This striking image, in which death and life coexist, stands for tribal survivance in the midst of perpetual threats.

Unresolved Traumatic Grief

The trauma of Native Americans, according to Cynthia Wesley-Esquimaux and Magdalena Smolewski, is cumulative. The first one is physical, caused by mass murder and infectious diseases. The second one is economic, caused by the violation of their stewardship of the land. The third one is cultural, caused by their compulsive Christianization and prohibition of local belief systems. The fourth one is social, caused by their displacement during colonial expansion that damaged families, altered gender roles, and diminished cultural values. The last one is psychological, caused by their marginalization and impoverishment on their own lands (6). This cumulative trauma is stored in the collective memory of Native Americans; it is recollected in oral traditions, as in stories and songs, and transmitted from one generation to the next. Forgetting traumatic events seems impossible; they keep haunting the minds of survivors who continually relive the past through fragmented memories, hallucinations, and nightmares. The denial of mourning rights for almost a century led to the inability of many generations to resolve their traumatic grief (Brave Heart and DeBruyn 60). A federal law in 1883 prohibited the practice of Native American mourning ceremonies that were performed for centuries to release the burden of sorrow; the ban lasted until 1978 with the promulgation of the American Indian Religious Freedom Act.

To heal their unresolved traumatic grief, Native Americans believe in the healing power of the word through chants and stories. Nanapush recounts the way he saved his own life through stories during the epidemic, "During the year of sickness, when I was the last one left, I saved myself by starting a story. [...] I could hardly keep moving my lips. But I did continue and recovered. I got well by talking. Death could not get a word in edgewise, grew discouraged, and traveled on" (Erdrich 46). This testimony illustrates the healing power of storytelling in the Native American worldview, as Nanapush believes in the power of words to save from the clutches of death.

In another instance, when Fleur contracts tuberculosis, the sanitary agency imposes a quarantine on her and orders the burning of her house to eradicate the disease-causing germs. In so doing, they would metaphorically destroy her because she embodies the ancestral knowledge of tribal medicine. However, Nanapush comes to her rescue to ward off the "invisible sickness" through the power of chants and stories, and in this act, he saves not only the girl, but also the legacy of tribal medicine. Later, when faced with Lulu's severe frostbite, the physician proposes an amputation and asks Father Damien "to reason with the fool." Nanapush resolutely turns down the solution, saying, "You were a butterfly, a flash of wit and fire, a blur of movement who could not keep still. Saving you the doctor's way would kill you" (168). He believes that the girl's vibrant spirit would not cope with this radical treatment, and he takes it upon himself to support her healing journey. He devotes countless hours to bathing her feet in water and pickling salt, employing cleansing smoke and weaving narratives of healing to accompany her through the long and dark nights until she regains the ability to walk.

Conclusion

In Erdrich's *Tracks*, the assault of infectious diseases almost decimated Native American populations, and in conjunction, Manifest Destiny and broken treaties literally disregarded their sovereignty. Nanapush and Fleur, the tribal shamans, are the only survivors of a community exterminated by virgin soil epidemics, but they have inherited the gift of healing and the knowledge of herbs. The novel is a narrative of "survivance" (survival/endurance); it is "more than survival, more than endurance or mere response," but "an active repudiation of dominance, tragedy, and victimry" (Vizenor 15). It emphasizes the active presence of Indigenous people in contrast to the stereotype of the Vanishing Indian, serving as acts of resistance against the master narratives of mainstream culture.

2 The Double Helix of Medical Knowledge Systems in Amitav Ghosh's *The Calcutta Chromosome: A Novel of Fevers, Delirium, and Discovery*

Introduction

Indian writer Amitav Ghosh's *The Calcutta Chromosome: A Novel of Fevers, Delirium, and Discovery* (1995) is a combination of medical thriller, historical fiction, and science fiction. Its central theme is the history of medicine and scientific research in India, with a focus on colonial medicine in the figure of Ronald Ross, a British physician who won the Nobel Prize in Physiology or Medicine (1902) for his work on malaria.[12] In so doing, the novel reflects on the broader history of imperialism and its reliance on science to accommodate its political and economic interests. Drawing from his expertise as an anthropologist, Ghosh challenges the dominance of one worldview by using the metaphor of the chromosome. Its double helix can be the symbol of a unifying entity for the Euro-America-centric and Indigenous knowledge systems.[13] He shares his ambition for a medical pluralism that considers medicine beyond the divisions of Western/non-Western and modern/ traditional. He might have found inspiration in the study of medical pluralism in the late 1970s to early 1980s when anthropologists compared medical systems and emphasized the value of syncretism[14] (Khalikova 4).

Ronald Ross: Figure of Scientific Imperialism

Ronald Ross (see figure 8) can be considered, in a way, as one of the health humanists of his time; he was not only a physician, but also a poet and a novelist. It is

---

[12] Prior to British colonization, cases of malaria were prevalent in India. However, the situation worsened after the expansion of irrigation systems, coupled with the industrialization of urban centers like Calcutta and Bombay. This expansion was not attended by substantial hygienic conditions, leading to an increase in the incidence of malaria (Packard 87–88).
[13] I make a deliberate shift from using the adjective "Western" as a broad, geographically unbounded conception of knowledge, to using "Euro-America-centered" as only two distinct geographical locations.
[14] See Kristine Krause et al. "Turning Therapies: Placing Medical Diversity." *Medical Anthropology*, vol. 33, no. 1, 2014, pp. 1–5.

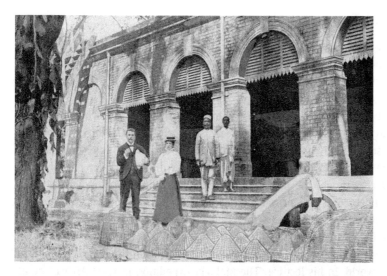

Figure 8: Ronald Ross and his Wife (1898) (Public domain image, reproduced from the CDC)

believed, however, that Ross "had no predisposition to medicine" (CDC) because, despite his aspiration to pursue a writing career, his father arranged for his enrollment at St Bartholomew's Hospital Medical College in London (Apte 68). His medical education was, therefore, not wholehearted, and he predominantly devoted his time to creative writing and music composition. In his account of the circumstances surrounding the discovery of the Anopheles mosquito species as the carrier of human malaria, Ross writes in his *Memoirs*, "Now, as if in answer, some Angel of Fate must have met one of my three 'mosquito men' in his leisurely perambulations and must have put into his hand a bottle of mosquito larvæ" (221). His writing is a fusion of scientific knowledge and Christian faith where both logic and belief are of equal importance, and his lyrical prose brims with religious imagery such as the mysterious "Angel of Fate." He keeps, however, the identities of the "Angel of Fate" and the "mosquito men" concealed, implying the probable involvement of occult forces.

Ross celebrated the discovery of the malaria parasite in 1897 by sending a poem to his wife, presently engraved on a commemorative stone at the Presidency General Hospital in Calcutta, and quoted by Ghosh as an epigraph to *The Calcutta Chromosome: A Novel of Fevers, Delirium, and Discovery:*

> This day relenting God
> Hath placed within my hand
> A wondrous thing; and God

> Be praised. At His command,
> Seeking His secret deeds
> With tears and toiling breath,
> I find thy cunning seeds,
> O million-murdering Death. (2)

In his Nobel Prize lecture in 1902, Ross exhibited a notable lack of modesty in the presentation of his discovery and imperialist rhetoric in his identification of malaria. He described the virus as the "gigantic ally of barbarism" that "strikes down not only the indigenous barbaric population but, with still greater certainty, the pioneers of civilization, the planter, the trader, the missionary and the soldier" (qtd. in B. Ghosh 264). He glorified the role of Western civilization in taming the perceived savagery of the "barbaric" populations. He embraced the imperialist rhetoric of his time, by virtue of which Western powers had a moral duty, known as the "civilizing mission," to bestow their light on the less developed regions of the world. In his lecture "The Malaria Expedition in West Africa," he asserts that "the success of Imperialism would depend largely upon the success of the microscope" (36). Ross' self-infatuated glorification of his discovery rests on the dissension between Western and other knowledge systems, as his speeches link scientific discovery with territorial expansion.

In his *Memoirs*, Ross presents his achievement as more glorious than the discoveries of Christopher Columbus and other explorers. He writes, "I am sure that none of them would ever have embarked on so vast and stormy a sea, would ever have been a Columbus of so wild an adventure, would ever have shown – I will not say the patience, the passion, and the poetry – but the madness required to find that uncharted treasure island!" (227). The language and tone of this quote associate scientific discovery with imperialism, comparing mosquitoes to an "uncharted" territory waiting to be mapped by a valiant explorer like himself. Ross' imperialist discourse voices the belief in René Descartes' theory of dualism between the mind and the body, the Cartesian thinking of Western science that views the world as a collection of separate, predictable parts governed by fixed laws. In the same logic, Michel Foucault argues that power operates through, and is sustained by, knowledge systems and discourses[15]. Power produces knowledge, shaping what is consid-

---

[15] In "Indigenous Knowledge Foundations for First Nations," Marie Battiste uses the concept of "cognitive imperialism" (9) to denounce the Euro-American alteration of chronological records and the negation of non-European knowledges, such as Mayan, Hindu, and Arabic. She also observes the Europeanization of the names of scientists and the appropriation of their work; she provides the example of the comet identified by the Chinese over 2,500 years ago and wrongly credited to Edmund Haley (2).

ered valid and acceptable, and conversely, knowledge serves as a form of power that grants authority to control individuals (119). As a consequence, Cartesian science has marginalized Indigenous knowledge systems as superstitious or occult practices.

Western vs. Occult Medical Knowledge

Ghosh was probably influenced by Franz Hartmann, a German physician and occultist interested in secret mystical knowledge, also known for his writings on esoteric healing and alternative medicine. In his book, *Occult Science in Medicine* (1893), he calls attention to the wealth of ancient medical knowledge that was categorized as occult. Employing Ross' *Memoirs* as a recurring motif, the narrative unfolds around the pursuit of the "cunning seeds" responsible for the malaria parasite described as the *"million murdering Death"* (Ghosh 40). To do so, the author blends fact and fiction to rewrite the story behind the occult discovery of malaria.

In *The Calcutta Chromosome: A Novel of Fevers, Delirium, and Discovery*, Murugan, medical archivist, argues that Ross had no inclination towards medicine, and that suddenly, he became vested in malaria research. He describes him as "a real huntin', fishin', shootin', colonial type, like in the movies; plays tennis and polo and goes pig-sticking; good looking guy, thick moustache, chubby pink cheeks" (51). Murugan attributes Ross' achievement to a combination of fortunate speculation, Indigenous knowledge appropriation, and self-assurance. He sardonically says, "one morning he gets out of bed and finds he's been bitten by the science bug" (45), believing that he is conducting experiments on the malaria parasite, when in fact, he himself is the subject of experimentation involving the malaria parasite. Murugan believes that Ross functioned merely as a conduit for a secret subaltern agency specialized in traditional Indian medicine, which actually "discovered the manner in which malaria is conveyed by mosquitoes" (20). He bases his opinions on data compiled in the archives of LifeWatch, a non-profit organization headquartered in New York that acts as a global health consulting company and repository of data.

In one of the articles, Murugan uses the concept of "Other Mind" to signify the existence of mysterious individuals who have intentionally intervened in Ronald Ross' experiments, steering malaria research in specific directions while diverting attention from other directions. Mangala and Lutchman represent this occult, called counter-science in the novel. They are engaged in mysterious beliefs and practices with mystical or paranormal subjects. Their activity is characterized by its secretive nature, involving rituals, symbols, and practices that are not readily accessible or comprehensible to ordinary people. They explore realms of existence beyond the physical world and probe into spiritual and metaphysical aspects of reality. They have already discovered the mechanisms of malaria transmission, and they are investigating an enigmatic malaria chromosome, called the Calcutta chromosome, that has the potential to cure syphilis. The administration of this chromosome to humans is, however, hazardous as it results in neurological disorders. They hence believe that "the next big leap in their project will come from a mutation in the parasite," and they must "find a conventional scientist who'll give it a push" (92). The occultists surreptitiously communicate their knowledge about Malaria transmission to Ross, driven by the motif that global recognition of this discovery would unveil further variants and insights.

When Mangala has "reached a dead end," the solution is to provoke "another mutant." She knows that if she desires to bring about a specific kind of mutation, she can accomplish it by allowing things to be known. In her view, once the parasite "had been figured out, it would spontaneously mutate in directions that would take her work to the next step" (214). This explanation is based on her belief in reincarnation. The mystery in the occultists' action is that they could have claimed the discovery for themselves but prefer to attribute it to Ross. Antar, Murugan's colleague in New York, inquires about the reason why they do not attribute the research to themselves and win the Nobel Prize. In fact, the occultists "forget about diseases and cures and epidemiology and shit like that." What they are after is "much bigger," lying in "the ultimate transcendence of nature" (105). They must work secretly because, they believe, communicating would mean claiming to possess knowledge, which is the initial principle their counter-science rejects (88). The "impossibility of knowledge" (104) in this approach draws upon both postmodernist thought and Hindu philosophy by virtue of which acknowledging one's lack of complete knowledge is the initial step towards acquiring knowledge (Chambers 41–42). In Ghosh's novel, the counter-scientific group has outpaced orthodox medicine in research, identifying the female *anopheles* mosquito as the vector of malaria. The author suggests that the routes of science and medicine between Britain and India are not unidirectional as the proponents of the civilizing mission claim, but they involve a bidirectional exchange. The difference between the two sides is that "the one makes a great deal of clamour and show, the other is silent and not publicly known" (Hartmann 2). While Ross glorifies the discovery of the malaria parasite, Mangala silently works on moving its chromosome to the next stage in the treatment of syphilis.

The Double Helix of Knowledge Systems

The Calcutta Chromosome: A Novel of Fevers, Delirium, and Discovery is a postmodern novel that reflects Ghosh's "incredulity towards meta-narratives," using the words of French philosopher Jean-François Lyotard. The latter questions Western supremacy by asserting that its knowledge dominance through metanarratives, or grand narratives, claims universal and absolute truths, ignoring the existence of other forms of knowledge. He advocates the recognition of the plurality of knowledge systems because "scientific knowledge does not represent the totality of knowledge; it has always existed in addition to, and in competition and conflict with, another kind of knowledge" (7). Hence, Ghosh reflects the 1990s current of questioning the supremacy of the Western knowledge system and condemning its epistemic violence against Indigenous knowledge systems.

Gayatri Spivak draws partly on Foucault's study of the power/knowledge nexus to expose the "epistemic violence"[16] of colonialism whose dominant voice perpetuated systems of oppression by silencing marginalized others. She describes the ways in which one dominant knowledge system inflicts erasure upon other knowledge systems, imposing one group's worldview and devaluing alternative worldviews, thereby perpetuating power imbalances and reinforcing hegemony. Emphasizing the intersections of racism, sexism, and classism in this epistemic violence, Spivak calls for a counter-hegemonic commitment to decenter the privileged knowledge system, "unlearning" its supremacy, and opening up alternative ways of knowing (271–272). This seems to be Ghosh's enterprise in *The Calcutta Chromosome: A Novel of Fevers, Delirium, and Discovery.*

In the genetic symbolism of novel, the double helix[17] (see figure 9) can be interpreted as a metaphor for the fusion of Euro-America-centric and Indigenous knowledge systems. Just like the intertwined strands of a double helix, the two systems can unite to offer a comprehensive understanding of the world. In "The Chromosome as Concept and Metaphor in Amitav Ghosh's *The Calcutta Chromosome*," Julia Fendt considers that the metaphor of the chromosome calls "into question the

---

16 Boaventura de Sousa Santos uses the term "Epistemicide" to capture the dominant epistemic systems in the Global North and their hegemonic control over knowledge production in the Global South, and over Indigenous and immigrant populations residing in the Global North itself. See her *Epistemologies of the South: Justice against Epistemicide*. Paradigm Publishers, 2014.

17 The double helix refers to the DNA that is shaped like a twisted ladder. It is made up of two strands that are connected and wound around each other, forming a helix shape, like a twisted ladder; it carries genetic information and enables hereditary transmission of given traits. Beyond its scientific meaning, the double helix has become a symbolic representation of the essence of life and knowledge (Falco).

limits of knowledge as well as hierarchies and imbalances in knowledge production" (176). Murugan, in this sense, plays the role of the enzyme that decodes the DNA of the story to reveal the secret Calcutta chromosome. He says, "My part in this was to tie some threads together so that they could hand the whole package over in a neat little bundle some time in the future" (Ghosh 303). The "neat little bundle" metaphorically refers to the double helix, in which the helicase (an enzyme) unwinds and separates the two strands to expose the genetic information stored in the DNA.

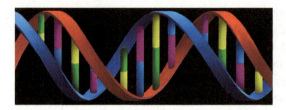

Figure 9: The Double Helix (free png)

Conclusion

Ghosh's *The Calcutta Chromosome: A Novel of Fevers, Delirium, and Discovery* is an archival novel about medical anthropology that tries to decolonize medical knowledge by incorporating Indigenous knowledge systems. At the literal level, it explores an aspect of the hidden histories of colonial medical research. At the metaphoric level, as the chromosome is a fundamental unit of genetic material, it stands for the complementarity between Euro-America-centric and Indigenous knowledge systems. Just as the chromosome carries vital genetic information within its structure, these knowledge systems have complementary perspectives to understand the complexity of the world. Each of the chromosomes possesses its own distinct wisdom, like the genetic code, that contributes to the understanding of human experience.

3 AIDS: "Accelerated Inner Development Syndrome" in Meja Mwangi's *Crossroads: The Last Plague*

Introduction

Crossroads: The Last Plague (1997) is Meja Mwangi's representation of a Kenyan society on the brink of extinction because of HIV/AIDS (Human Immunodeficiency Virus/Acquired Immunodeficiency Syndrome). It is set in a village called "Crossroads" where people must choose between fighting the epidemic and perishing. In a society that considers condoms as unmanly objects, Janet is a health educator who challenges social taboos to stop the epidemic progression. Her determination eventually leads to a positive aspect symbolized by the repentance of her AIDS-affected husband who simultaneously experiences a positive form of AIDS (Accelerated **I**nner **D**evelopment **S**yndrome). It is a condition of life review, enhanced spirituality, and exceptional generosity in the face of terminal disease. The play on words demonstrates with poignant lucidity that within the deepest affliction lies the potential to impart moral lessons to the fragile human soul.

Reckless Responses to the Sweeping Epidemic

Meja Mwangi's *Crossroads: The Last Plague* is set amidst the backdrop of different sociopolitical issues; the events happen in a Kenyan village in the 1980s during Daniel arap Moi's dictatorship. The political corruption and repression affected the lives of ordinary Kenyans, chiefly those living in poverty. During that period, the effects of globalization became perceptible in Kenyan society, particularly among the youth. Chief among the issues of that period was the outbreak of the HIV/AIDS epidemic, as well as the fear and stigma that surrounded it. The significance of this topic cannot be overstated in the field of global health humanities, especially in relation to an Africa novel. In the latest updates on HIV/AIDS statistics (2023), the World Health Organization indicates that the epidemic continues to pose an important global health challenge, with 40.1 million AIDS-affected persons claimed around the world, two-thirds of whom in the African Region. This highlights the urgent need for global health to raise more awareness in this continent where the burden is most concentrated.

Reading a novel like Mwangi's *Crossroads: The Last Plague* can serve as a reminder of the ongoing efforts required to combat the epidemic. It provides a mordant review of the widespread ignorance about HIV and its transmission; the characters do not protect themselves and their partners because they simply do not understand how the virus is transmitted or because their male chauvinism emboldens them to take risks. The consequences of both causes are tragic as the epidemic takes a heavy toll on the community. To make things worse, the villagers do not look for guidance regarding virus transmission routes and prevention methods owing to the taboo nature of the issue. There is no radio station in the village; the single phone booth is inoperative and squatted by a beggar. The only source of information is Uncle Mark who peruses outdated newspapers delivered by the sole bus that traverses the village. The other vehicles that visit the place are the ones that carry the lifeless bodies of the sons and daughters who left it in pursuit of better opportunities somewhere else. These are "ox-wagons and donkey carts, loaded with coffins and hung with red flags, dutifully delivered their cold burdens to the gaping holes that awaited them in every village and in every hamlet and in every homestead all over Crossroads" (Mwangi 21). This passage vividly captures the somber atmosphere surrounding the procession of vehicles that transport coffins and mourners; the description of the vehicles as heavy laden conveys not only the death toll, but also the emotional weight endured by the families.

The socioeconomic situation is alarming, as most businesses have gone bankrupt; the act of digging graves has replaced tending to the land, transforming the once productive cultivation of cassava into the somber burial of human beings. The narrator poignantly explains the worrying scale of the disease; it is "turning everything upside down, buffeting communities and shattering hopes and dreams, crushing minds and spirits and leaving behind only emptiness and despair" (4). In this apocalyptic tone, the imminent threat of infection is sweeping everyone away; people refrain from making long-term plans in their bleak outlook for the future.

In African culture, as in many parts of the world[18], there exists a prevailing belief that risk-taking, even in the face of deadly viruses, is a defining feature of intrepidity and masculinity. As a result, men may be reluctant to adopt preventive measures, such as using condoms, in order to satisfy the perceived expectations of masculinity. The concept of "Young Male Syndrome (YMS)" is used to denote elevated rates of risk-taking among "the male population between the ages of 15–35 years, the time when intrasexual competition is the strongest" (Wilson 59). In *Crossroads: The Last Plague*, therefore, Mwangi reflects the global concern of

---

18 Will H. Courtenay studies the same risk-taking behaviors among American men. See his article "Engendering Health: A Social Constructionist Examination of Men's Health Beliefs and Behaviors." *Psychology of Men & Masculinity*, vol. 1, no. 1, 2000, pp. 4–15. www.psycnet.apa.org/record/2000-13038-001

men's risk-taking behaviors in relation to HIV/AIDS. The author lays blame, to a considerable degree, on the unbridled libido of men who associate masculinity with risk-taking. A "total" man, in the local culture, is one who does not use condoms because they decrease the pleasure of sexual contact; he is also one who has many wives and/or sex partners. Broker, an AIDS-affected character who used to hold firmly to these beliefs before his contamination, tells his wife Janet that it is not easy to convince "total" men that a condom does not affect their virility. He acknowledges the challenge of persuading Crossroads men, who are stubborn and resistant to change, that using a condom does not diminish their sexual prowess; he admits his own errors and commits to fighting prevalent misconceptions.

In the local tradition of Crossroads, when a man dies, his brother inherits his wife to protect the orphans from the ill-treatment of a non-relative stepfather. In this case, Janet seeks to dissuade her brother-in-law, Kata, from marrying his brother's widow because the latter succumbed to AIDS. Supported by the elders, and considering himself as a custodian of traditions, Kata refuses the "unmanly" action of forsaking his brother's widow and orphans. Moreover, he adamantly rejects the use of condoms as a preventive measure, even Grandmother advises Janet to let him confront his destiny as a man. The name Kata, on that matter, is the equivalent of "the stubborn one" in Swahili, standing for his "bullheadedness" and refusal to change in defiance of the greatest adversities. In reference to that, the metaphor of the bull is recurrent in the novel to convey not only virility and power, but also the cruelty and destruction of men whose unrestrained sexual energies are threatening the whole community. Even elderly males consider themselves "old bulls," striving to maintain their social status by proudly exhibiting their sexual vitality. When Broker becomes a sober man, his mother regrets the "bull" he used to be and laments the "goat" he has become. Ironically, she laments his departure from the expected norms of masculinity, reflecting her blind conformity to the patriarchal mindset.

Women's Vulnerability to the Epidemic

Of major concern in the novel, as in the field of global health, is masculine risk-raking and gender-related vulnerability since "Epidemiological evidence suggests unacceptably high HIV prevalence and incidence rates among women. A multitude of factors increase women's vulnerability to HIV acquisition, including biological, behavioral, socioeconomic, cultural and structural risks" (Ramjee and Daniels 1). At the biological level, women have mucosal or hormonal factors that augment their vulnerability to HIV. At the behavioral level, societal norms and gender inequalities undermine women's ability to negotiate safe sexual practices, especially in patriarchal African societies. Regarding socioeconomic factors, women suffer from higher rates of illiteracy, poverty, and economic dependence. Cultural and societal norms equally play a major role in shaping their vulnerability, such as stigma and discrimination that can dissuade them from seeking HIV-related counseling and screening. Finally, structural factors include the limited availability of healthcare services and the lack of legal protection. The interaction of these factors contribute to the status of African women as the most vulnerable individuals to the epidemic, necessitating appropriate interventions for their rescue.

In *Crossroads: The Last Plague*, Kata's wife accepts, without resistance, his marriage with his late brother's widow; she is even annoyed when Janet asks her to prevent him from doing so. She admits that she cannot even ask him to use condoms since, as a "total man," he disregards any counsel offered by women. Crossroads women, to use Fanon's word, have "epidermalized" their inferiority (*Black Skin* 4) to such an extent that they no longer think whether their dignity is being violated or their lives are being at risk. The grandmother, stunned by Janet's words, yells, "What are you telling your sister now? You know she cannot leave her husband" (Mwangi 56); she means that a woman cannot afford her living, and that she is a possession he "bought and paid for completely" (52). In addition to her conviction that the dowry makes a woman her husband's possession, the grandmother persistently reprimands Janet for her abominable call for protective condoms and contraceptive pills.

Janet is the only unwavering female fighter in the village, and she is treated as a pariah for that, but her economic independence allows her to protest. She has been separated from Broker, her former husband, for more than ten years because of his engagement in extramarital affairs and contamination by the HIV virus. Despite facing derogatory remarks from women and receiving advances from men, she remains resolute in her decision to remain unmarried. Even when Broker returns, expressing remorse, she firmly rejects any possibility of reconciliation. The other women in the village, who are socioeconomically dependent on their husbands, cannot afford to defy their husbands. Janet is even regarded as a prostitute for not having a man who rules her actions; her sister tells her, "We have husbands. We are not prostitutes" (53). Living in a patriarchal African community, women like Janet can be despised and even treated as "prostitutes" because they disrupt the established order of ancestral customs and gender roles; they are usually considered as a threat to social stability. Janet is, as the only female fighter in a patriarchal society, disdainfully treated as "condom lady" and "shameless woman." The narrator explains, "Some say she was a creature from mad women's hell, an angry spirit sent back to torment Crossroads men." That "was why her husband had run off with another woman. What she needed now, they said with drunker fervour, was an ox trainer, someone to whip her back to womanhood" (61).

Mzee Musa believes she needs a man to make her pregnant, the only way to transform her into a "proper" woman; the action of impregnating women is so regarded as a weapon for subduing their sexuality and subjugating their minds.

Eventually, the sight of AIDS-stricken bodies in a book shared by Janet instills a deep sense of fear in a woman called Hanna who ventures to defy her husband, telling him about the risks of his promiscuous behavior. Under the effect of panic, he agrees to use condoms on the condition that she keeps the secret for fear of him being considered unmanly. The shocking images in the book ultimately have the same effect on Kata, and he finally concedes to using condoms. These instances, which prove that a picture is worth a thousand words, also reflect the men's deep anxiety about losing their social perception of virility, probably more than their fear of losing their lives. Deplorably, Hanna discovers her HIV-positive status, contracted from her husband who in turn contracted it from his other wife. In her painful revelation, the guiltless woman bears the burden of her husband's polygamy, sanctioned by ingrained cultural beliefs surrounding masculinity and femininity. The narrator observes that in their relation with the epidemic, the villagers mistakenly think they are safe because they are not involved in extramarital affairs. Hanna's case reveals the reality that even within the sacred institution of marriage, engaging in sexual relations cannot assure protection against HIV infection.

Rational Responses to the Sweeping Epidemic

As an official health educator appointed by the government to face the deeply rooted taboos that favor the progression of the epidemic, Janet gathers her inner strength to undertake the noble task of educating people about safe sex, but she faces humiliation from both men and women who view the distribution of condoms as a shameful act. Undeterred by reprimands, she bravely confronts her adversaries' ignorance and carelessness, and her determination shines a ray of hope amidst an otherwise desolate landscape. Shame, she believes, lies on the other side that leads to the infection of innocent individuals with HIV and the marginalization of AIDS-stricken others. She calls attention to the repercussions of shame on the spread of the virus; because it is a taboo, people do not seek help and diagnostic testing, and in so doing, shame becomes a barrier to the fight against the epidemic.

It is beyond question that education plays a crucial role in the novel as the vehicle of change; by imparting knowledge and raising awareness among the population, it becomes a catalyst for transformative action. As a "responsible educator," Jane believes that, "without her teaching, the future the teachers claimed they prepared the pupils for would never be realized. This was why it was necessary to teach family life education in their schools" (342). As some characters ultimately learn from her about the disease, they take measures to protect themselves and their loved ones, using condoms and limiting the number of their partners. Janet's mission, in the narrator's view, is to fight against men who believe that using a condom is comparable to sleeping with gumboots or having a bath fully clothed. This reflection encapsulates some African men's perspective on masculinity and resistance to condoms; the comparison of wearing a condom to wearing gumboots to bed or taking a bath fully dressed reflects their belief that using protection diminishes their pleasure and undermines their perceived virility. For Janet, overcoming such deeply ingrained attitudes is more than just an obligation; it is a quixotic determination to fight long-standing beliefs and cultural norms. Though her intentions may be honorable, her approach to the difficult struggle against the epidemic is marked by immaturity. Her efforts to distribute free condoms to the villagers initially go unnoticed until Broker returns home; only in collaboration with him could the condom campaign yield results.

Life Review and Accelerated Inner Development Syndrome (AIDS)

Mwangi's *Crossroads: The Last Plague* represents an interesting response to HIV/AIDS through AIDS as an "**A**ccelerated **I**nner **D**evelopment **S**yndrome," a concept borrowed from John Masterson's *John Mordaunt: Facing up to AIDS as Told to John Masterson* (1989). It denotes a condition in which an individual experiences intense spiritual or psychological transformation, caused by various factors such as life-threatening disease, traumatic events, and near-death experiences. It is characterized by a sense of connection to oneself and others, as well as a deeper awareness of one's thoughts and emotions. In fact, even though AIDS-affected individuals may experience mood changes, anxiety, and depression because of their fear of the disease and death, they may also develop an understanding of the world and their place in it. This may result in detachment from material possessions and need for self-redemption.

Broker, who was living away from his family for many years, returns to Crossroads with the belief that his newfound wealth would ensure Janet's acceptance of him back into her life, but her gained material, intellectual, and emotional independence empower her to refuse. The grandmother believes Janet should forgive Broker because he is a "total" man, capable of providing for the family regardless of his adulterous past and contagious condition. Knowing that his days of seducing women are behind him, Broker resorts to using his financial status to assert his masculinity. Despite Janet's rejection of living with him, Broker makes an effort to be attentive to their children. He frequently collects them from school and takes them into leisure activities to make up for a lost time; sadly, his efforts to be a good father are interrupted when he passes away before nurturing a meaningful bond with them. Before drawing his last breath, Broker builds a fuel-filling station that invites car drivers to the desolate village; he offers a new service of selling the very condoms that Janet previously failed to distribute free of charge, attracting unprecedented interest in their use. While it may be perceived as unusual, this fact stands firm in the patriarchal mentality; the rejection of free condoms, proposed by a woman, reveals deeply rooted gender dynamics. In male-dominated societies, men are the providers and decision-makers while women need to conform to their submissive and nurturing roles. Janet's earlier distribution of condoms is, in this sense, dismissed as a threat to male dominance.

The idea of Broker, inspired by his own masculinity and knowledge about the mindset of his fellows, is to sell condoms instead of giving them away at no cost. He is certain that no man would purchase a condom and dispose of it. His reflection, be it ever so simple, reflects an underlying belief that when individuals invest their own money in purchasing some goods, they are less likely to discard them unused. His assumption that attaching a monetary value to condoms has indeed promoted their usage and contributed to safer sexual practices in *Crossroads*. Broker further engages in journalistic activism to raise awareness about the multiple challenges that hinder the integration of safer sexual practices within the community:

> He told the journalist of the poverty of the people, the conditions that rendered the community incapable of affording the most basic hygiene and medicine, let alone latex condoms.
>
> He talked of the ignorance that shackled the people to the earth like beasts of burden and the illiteracy that made it impossible for the community to understand Aids, and its potential for annihilation. (391)

The socioeconomic conditions, as it were, create a fertile terrain for the rampant spread of HIV/AIDS. Above all is the pervasive poverty that renders unattainable basic hygiene practices and access to essential medicines, let alone the usage of condoms for safe sexual practices. Ignorance correspondingly dampens people's understanding of HIV transmission and its harrowing consequences.[19]

Broker personifies the disease-afflicted but resilient individual who defies despair by embracing his limited time with altruism; his amassed material wealth

---

[19] To have an idea about the underlying causes of the frenzied spread of HIV in Africa more than any other place in the world, see Helen Epstein's *The Invisible Cure: Africa, the West, and the Fight against AIDS*. Farrar, Straus and Giroux, 2007.

finds purpose in nourishing the aspirations of his soul. To satisfy his philanthropic yearnings, he spends his time "surveying Crossroads, assessing old buildings and making plans for their restoration. He had enough plans for a whole lifetime of rebuilding" (209). For instance, he shows his benevolence towards the beggar by giving him not only subsistence through money, but also dignity through words. He also pays Head Faru's debt and contributes to the restoration of the church roof. Broker decides to dedicate the revenues generated from the condom shop to supporting the intergenerational center he calls "Janet Broker Home for Orphans and old Folk," in honor of his wife for whom he expresses his repentance and admiration. His wise approach reaps substantial rewards as Janet, despite her previous refusal, feels compassion towards him.

In psychotherapy, reviewing one's life assists elderly individuals and younger ones facing the inevitability of death to deal with unresolved issues in their lives. The aim is, according to psychiatrist and gerontologist Robert Butler, to cope with their fears in the here and now, a principle he calls "the therapeutic use of 'presentness'" (the presence of the past in the present). He posits, "Life review is characterized by the progressive return to consciousness of past experiences and, particularly, the resurgence of unresolved conflicts for reexamination and reintegration. If the reintegration is successful, such reminiscence can give new significance and meaning to life and prepare the person for death by mitigating fear and anxiety" (203). Through life review, the individual can "let off steam," to be liberated from their negative feelings related to the regrets of the past, the dissatisfactions of the present, and the anxieties of the future; this is made possible in the presence of human touch from relatives and friends. In his study of life review, Butler proves to be an early health humanities scholar. In the epigraph to one of his most quoted texts, "Prologue or Introduction to Life Review" (written in 1963), he uses a verse from William Cowper's "Task" (1784), *"Mem'ry's pointing wand, that calls the past to our exact review"* (203), to illustrate the power of "presentness." Butler not only proves his interdisciplinary openness but yet again, the relevance of literature in the deepest medical reflections. He equally refers to art historian Bernard Berenson to explain the "life-enhancing experiences" that make "life a work of art," and that despite the dim situation, there is "still the opportunity for a sensuous appreciation of life" (qtd. in Achenbaum 19). Life review thus becomes a therapeutic and artistic chance for enlightenment and redemption.

Broker's benevolence in *Crossroads: The Last Plague* arises from his deep need to redefine existence and infuse it with significance, redeeming the errors of his past and nourishing his soul. Beyond the literal sense of a man who acts as an intermediary in financial transactions, Broker's name has meaningful connotations in the sense that "broker" can stand for a "mediator" or "peacemaker" who facilitates negotiations between Janet and the community, mainly the masculine community. The word is also close to "broken," suggesting the fragmentation caused by a life-threatening disease, but it also implies a negotiation of transformation as part of an "Accelerated Inner Development Syndrome." He harvests the respect of everyone so that, upon his departure, all those whose lives he has affected feel a deep sense of loss. His expanded spirituality empowers him to embrace his remaining time with purpose, rendering him strong in the face of death's inevitability.

Conclusion

Mwangi's *Crossroads: The Last Plague* casts light on the importance of education in raising awareness about the prevention and spread of HIV/AIDS; it also stresses the importance of community-based responses to it in the face of stigma and taboo. In the mouth of his narrator, the elimination of taboos involves discussions on practicing safe sex, using condoms, and limiting the number of partners. The bright side of the story lies in the rise of hope amidst despair, as Broker develops "Accelerated Inner Development Syndrome," characterized by an intense transformation of subjectivity. His past serves as a cautionary tale for young individuals who engage in unprotected sex, and his present offers a lesson to those afflicted by a devastating illness to find peace at the dusk of life.

Part III: **Mental Disorders in the Global Anglophone Novel**

1 Lingering Wounds of Maternal Abandonment in Toni Morrison's *A Mercy*

Introduction

Toni Morrison's *A Mercy* (2008) unfurls as a poignant addition to her historical sagas about slavery. Set in the late 17th century during the formative years of slavery, it probes into the somber facets of colonial America to explore the critical themes of trauma and resilience. The protagonists, burdened by their individual tales of distress, embark on introspective journeys into the depths of their pasts, seeking to confront the enduring scars of maternal abandonment that hinder their ability to find solace in the present. Helped by their African American healing knowledge and the redemptive power of the word, their dormant pain resurfaces, yet emerges the aspiration for a more peaceful time ahead.

The Trauma of Maternal Abandonment

The trauma of abandonment refers to the psychological distress experienced by individuals who have been deserted or rejected by someone significant in their lives. It can occur in various contexts, such as parental abandonments or romantic relationship breakups. Individuals may develop feelings of insecurity, low self-esteem, and fear of rejection; they might never trust anyone again or maintain healthy relationships. Abandonment trauma can also lead to emotional numbing and persistent feelings of grief; some individuals may exhibit self-destructive behaviors, such as self-mutilation or substance abuse.

Maternal abandonment is a leitmotif in Morrison's fiction, in which mothers commit infanticide, as in *Sula* and *Beloved*, or abandon their child, as in *Jazz* and *A Mercy*. Many scarred characters in these novels are women since, for Morrison, "to be female in this place is to be an open wound that cannot heal. Even if scars form, the festering is ever below" (*A Mercy* 193). Many of Morrison's novels are related to the institution of slavery that, in essence, connotes an abandonment of humanity as it strips the slaveholders of their mercy and the enslaved of their dignity. In the context of slavery, women are considered doubly oppressed; first, by the patriarchal system, and second, by the slave systems. The black female characters in Morrison's novels often bear deep-seated physical and emotional wounds inflicted by the oppressive society in which they exist. These women are often victims of segregation, humiliation, and rape; they occasionally resort to violence, verbal or physical, to protect themselves from further suffering. This victimization is often directed at the closest family and community members.

Morrison's *A Mercy* explores the black female slave's affliction in America by weaving the narratives of vulnerable mothers and forsaken children. When reading *A Mercy*, one cannot help but draw parallels with *Beloved* (1987), the masterpiece in which Morrison also explores the theme of maternal abandonment. Beloved's mother, like Florens' mother, abruptly severs the parental bond in a desperate attempt to shield her daughter from the horrors of slavery. What Florens and Beloved call an act of *abandonment*, the mothers call an act of *mercy*. The back-cover blurb of *A Mercy* indicates: "A Mercy reveals what lies beneath the surface of slavery. But at its heart, it is the ambivalent, disturbing story of a mother who casts off her daughter in order to save her and of a daughter who may never exorcise that abandonment. Acts of mercy may have unforeseen consequences." Morrison's mothers hence assert their maternal role in ways that pose a complex challenge to comprehension with contemporary moral standards.

In Morrison's *A Mercy*, "a minha mãe," "My Mother" in Portuguese, perceives in Jacob Vaark a mercy she does not find in other slaveholders; she sees "no animal in his heart" (191) compared to other slaveholders who have raped her and started coveting her daughter's maturing body. She decides to give him Florens to treat her "as a human child" (195), and therefore save her from being sexually abused at the hands of merciless slaveholders. Nevertheless, due to the absence of any explanation behind the mother's decision, the daughter internalizes the belief that her mother relinquished her. She understands the act of her mother as prioritizing her newborn brother, causing severe damage to her self-worth and hindering her ability to foster human ties.

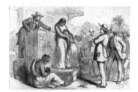

Figure 10: Slave Auction in the Deep South (circa 1850) in Edmund Ollier's *Cassell's History of the United States* (1874–77). (Public domain image reproduced from "Slavery Images: A Visual Record of the African Slave Trade in the Early African Diaspora." www.slaveryimages.org/s/slaveryimages/item/1878

Upon her arrival to Vaark's plantation, Florens is unable to speak, an indication of the deep-seated trauma she carries within, and she jealously imagines her mother nursing her hungry brother. She says, "forever and ever. Me watching, my mother listening, her baby boy on her hip. Senhor is not paying the whole amount he owes to Sir. Sir saying he will take instead the woman and the girl, not the baby boy and the debt is gone. A minha mãe begs no. Her baby boy is still at her breast. *Take the girl*, she says, *my daughter*, she says. *Me. Me*" (Morrison, *A Mercy* 7, emphasis added). The mother's words are constantly reenacted, like haunting Florens' mind. She suffers from dissociated consciousness which, as Bessel A. Van der Kolk and Onno van der Hart explain, "reflects a horizontally layered model of mind: when a subject does not remember a trauma, its 'memory' is contained in an alternate stream of consciousness, which may be subconscious or dominate consciousness, e.g., during traumatic reenactments" (168). Maternal abandonment, therefore, creates a rupture in the mother-child bond that disrupts Florens' process of identity formation and the establishment of a sense of self. The mother, who is supposed to provide love and care, becomes a synonym of rejection. This disruption of the maternal presence creates a sense of disorientation, with contradictory feelings of longing for the absent mother and feelings of anger, sadness, and fear. This ambivalence creates a deep-seated emotional conflict that defines the character's later experiences.

Florens is too young to interpret the complex dimensions of her mother's traumatic decision, and she lives the rest of her life with what Morrison describes in *Jazz* (1992) as "mother hunger hit her like a hammer" (3). She feels, however, that her mother wants to tell her a message, of which she is unable to make sense; her trauma is acting like a distorting filter through which she perceives human relations. Vaark gives the motherless Florens as a present to his childless wife Rebekka, a present the latter does not seem to accept. It is Lina, the Native American servant, who serves as a surrogate mother for Florens; they "slept together, bathed together, ate together and Lina made clothes and tiny shoes from rabbit skin for Florens" (Morrison, *A Mercy* 124), indicating a form of solidarity between Native Americans and African Americans in the early years of the nation. When the blacksmith enters Florens' life, Lina worries about the outcome because "she was struck down with another sickness much longer lasting and far more lethal" (127). Falling in love initially compensates Florens' feeling of abandonment; she tells him, "You are my protection. Only you" (81). When she goes to his house, she meets an orphaned boy who clings to a doll for comfort. While the Blacksmith is away, Florens looks after the boy, yet she harbors a growing resentment towards him, fearing that the Blacksmith would prioritize the boy over her. She says, "I worry as the boy steps closer to you [...] As if he is your future. Not me" (136). In an unfortunate turn of events, she fractures the boy's arm while trying to hush him, leading the Blacksmith to drive her out of his house and his life.

Lina equally suffers from the trauma of abandonment, coupled with a pang of survivor guilt. Insinuating to Jeffery Amherst's "germ warfare" against Native

Americans through smallpox-infected blankets, she recounts the loss of her tribe to the "blankets they could neither abide nor abandon." In this tragic episode, she continues, "Infants fell silent first, and even as their mothers heaped earth over their bones, they too were pouring sweat and limp as maize hair" (54). Yet, when Lina sets foot on Vaark's plantation, her survivor guilt subsides "with her vow never to betray or abandon anyone she cherished" (57). Owing to her intense fear of being devoid of familial support, Lina willingly submits to being "cleansed" by Presbyterian rescuers, only to face abandonment again.

Sorrow, described as a "mongrel," is another character who suffers from "mother hunger," being the unique survivor of a shipwreck in which her family perished. She cannot remember the traumatic event, apart from being pulled to the shore by whales. The narrator relates, "Now the memories of the ship, the only home she knew, seemed as stolen as its cargo [...]. Even the trace of Captain was dim" (117). The presence of memory gaps is indicative of Sorrow's dissociative disorder because traumatic memories are frequently relegated to a distinct compartment within the mind. Twin, her imaginary alter ego and symptom of her divided self, enters her existence when she opens her eyes in the shipwrecked vessel; he turns into her "safety, her entertainment, her guide" (119). In *The Divided Self: An Existential Study in Sanity and Madness,* Ronald Laing explains that the schizoid individual cannot nurture relationships with real-life people, but can relate with "depersonalized persons, to phantoms of his own phantasies (imagos), perhaps to things, perhaps to animals" (77). Twin is a manifestation of Sorrow's schizoid identity; he functions as a coping mechanism that enables her to survive in adversarial conditions. Laing adds that "the imagined advantages" of the divided self "are safety for the true self, isolation and hence freedom from others, self-sufficiency, and control" (75). Sorrow's reliance on a depersonalized relationship, for fear of genuine human relationships, is a living example of human resilience amidst maddening conditions. The girl is taken into the care of a sawyer's family, where his wife calls her Sorrow to reflect her orphaned soul, but she is repeatedly raped by his two sons. When she is sold to Vaark, she is pregnant at the tender age of eleven. Her initial encounter with motherhood is traumatic, as Lina throws the newborn into the river. The loss of the child exacerbates Sorrow's already fragile mental state, leading her to communicate with Twin more than ever before.

Mending the Mind within

In the case of Florens, Lina, and Sorrow, transformation becomes necessary to break the harmful cycle of traumatic reenactment; it can help them assimilate the painful memories into their cognitive frameworks, leading to personal growth.

Mental health requires that the child "experience a warm, intimate, and continuous relationship with his or her mother or mother-substitute in which both find satisfaction" (Bowlby 76). Through love and resilience, these characters can forge bonds that can heal their wounded souls. Essential to the healing process of these multiethnic American girls is the need to be treated with their traditional practices in their ancestral environments. Lina, for instance, embodies the conservationist spirit of Native Americans as she respects the sacred connections with the natural world and expresses her concern when Jacob Vaark fells trees to build his mansion. She also cures Rebekka Vaark by "piecing together scraps of what her mother had taught her before dying in agony" (Morrison, *A Mercy* 56), drawing upon her knowledge of medicinal herbs. She treats Rebekka with a mixture of mugwort, Saint-John's-wort, maidenhair, devil's bit, and periwinkle.

Another major healer in the novel is the blacksmith who has been commissioned to construct a fence for the newly constructed mansion. He masterfully treats Sorrow's smallpox infection with vinegar. The narrator provides evocative details:

> [...] he doused Sorrow's boils and the skin of her face and arms, sending her into spasms of pain. While the women sucked air and Sir frowned, the blacksmith heated a knife and slit open one of the swellings. They watched in silence as he tipped Sorrow's own blood drops between her lips. [...] Bit by bit, under the smithy's care and Florens' nursing, the boils shriveled, the welts disappeared and her strength returned. Now their judgment was clear: the blacksmith was a savior. (148–150)

With the blacksmith's healing knowledge and Florens' devoted nursing, Sorrow's boils decrease, her welts fade, and her vitality returns; all the witnesses understand that the blacksmith is a rescuer.

The blacksmith's healing knowledge represents the African American preservation of their ethnomedical traditions, transported from Africa along the slave route. In *Working Cures: Healing, Health, and Power on Southern Plantations*, Sharla Fett contends that in their countless encounters with enslaved laborers, slaveholders tried to destroy their souls and preserve their bodies, and in instances of slave resistance, physicians intervened, not to treat the body, but rather to exert control over it. She explores the various African American healing practices such as herbalism, conjuring, and midwifery that emerged as acts of resistance in the pre-Civil War South. When they were forcibly transported in the transatlantic slave trade, individuals from Igbo, Yoruba, Bambara, Kongo, and other African backgrounds transported their healing traditions to their new environment. They also drew upon the botanical knowledge of Native American medicine (1–2).

In *A Mercy*, an essential step in the girls' healing journey is the need to tell their stories. Trauma creates a speechless inner fight beyond direct representation;

it continues to haunt the individual until it is safely let out. In this case, Morrison's characters tell their stories as part of their therapeutic process. This approach is comparable to Narrative Exposure Therapy, which involves "an imaginal exposure" and is considered as a "treatment for trauma spectrum disorders in adult and child survivors of multiple stressors with complex trauma histories" (Schauer et al. 198). Stories therefore serve as therapeutic narratives for the traumatized characters in the novel, providing a potential for resilience to hold onto and a viewpoint after trauma to relate to.

In a significant manner, Florens often perceives her mother telling her an important message, but she cannot understand it; she says, "I will keep one sadness. That all the time I cannot know what my mother is telling me. Nor can she know what I am wanting to tell her" (Morrison, *A Mercy* 161). In the absence of her biological mother, Florens discovers a surrogate maternal figure in Lina who provides the nurturing she longs for; Lina acts as the storyteller who embraces her with the healing power of the word. She tells her stories with which she can identify, like the tale of bird eggs left by their mother to "hatch alone" (73) and the tale of the eagle that protected its eggs from man. The two of them spend "memorable nights, lying together, when Florens listened in rigid delight to Lina's stories [...]. Especially called for were the stories of mothers fighting to save their children from wolves and natural disasters" (72); the aim is to give her the different dimensions of motherhood with which she can identify.

In the same vein, Florens is fixated on "carving letters" and writing her story on the walls until "There is no more room in [the] room" (158). This is an instance of scriptotherapy, defined as the process of writing down a traumatic experience with a therapeutic purpose (Henke xii). Entering the room, she believes that sharing her story is alone capable of allowing her tears to flow freely. Despite her trauma of abandonment, it is important to conclude that Florens is not "a love-disabled girl" (Morrison, *A Mercy* 42). She ambivalently loves her absent-present mother; she sincerely loves Lina, her substitute mother, and she wholeheartedly loves the blacksmith, through whose love she feels free.

Sorrow is joyful at the prospect of new life developing within her; the "mother hunger" empowers her to preserve the fetus. She seeks the assistance of two indentured servants, named Will and Scully, to give birth. Of special significance is the disappearance of her "false self" (Laing 143), signifying the curative power of mothering. Committed to her newfound role as a mother, she recovers from her schizoid condition, and she gives herself a new name: "Complete." The narrator comments, "I am your mother" and "My name is Complete" (Morrison, *A Mercy* 134). This renaming signifies the transformative power of motherhood; with her newfound wholeness, Complete decides to escape from her bondage with Florens.

Eventually, the story of "a minha mãe" is also worth telling, and at the end of the novel, Morrison grants her the opportunity to let her voice be heard. She pleads that she is not "a soulless animal" (164). She relates the dehumanizing conditions of her deportation from her homeland as merchandise in the Atlantic slave trade. Before embarking, slaves were subjected to "culling," a selective removal of some individuals who do not correspond to the slave norms in terms of physical strength. To test their abilities, they "were made to jump high, to bend over, to open [their] mouths" (163). She explains that her distress and humiliation were so intense that she wished to die; she even "welcomed the circling sharks" since she "preferred their teeth to the chains" (162). In spite of being apart, the mother's yearning for Florens resonates through the poignant words: "hear a tua mãe [hear your mother]" (165).

Conclusion

In the context of slavery, therefore, the abandonment of a child can be seen as an act of mercy, albeit one that may be difficult to comprehend from a contemporary perspective. Slavery was an inherently dehumanizing system where enslaved individuals endured unspeakable violence. In such a situation, mothers who made the heart-wrenching decision to separate themselves from their children often did so out of a genuine desire to protect them from the horrors of enslavement. They recognized that a life of bondage, with its physical toil and psychological torment, was an unbearable fate for their children. By choosing to spare their children from a life of perpetual suffering, these mothers believed they were offering the ultimate act of mercy, liberating their children from the inhumane conditions they themselves were enduring. Lina, Florens, and Complete – representing Native American, African American, and mixed-heritage backgrounds – suffer from "mother hunger," while Jacob and Rebekka Vaark, as Euro-Americans, suffer from an unfulfilled desire for posterity. United in their shared yearning, they find solace within the walls of an ever-expanding mansion that symbolizes both the personal growth of everyone and the collective aspirations of the nation. In this portrayal, Morrison presents her optimistic vision of *E Pluribus Unum* (out of many, one) with diverse ethnic groups coexisting harmoniously within an American home, where benevolence bridges the racial divide and fosters peaceful coexistence.

2 Nervous Conditions in Tsitsi Dangarembga's Trilogy

Introduction

Africa is home to some of the world's most numerous hostilities, causing nervous conditions that find expression in literary works, and this chapter explores the nervous conditions of African women in Tsitsi Dangarembga's trilogy. Employing a host of Fanonist and Sartrean conceptual and theoretical tools, the author probes into the African woman's "epidermalization" of inferiority and the grim reality of the postcolonial condition whereby violence "detoxifies" the (formerly) colonized. The author was born in 1959 in Zimbabwe (then called Rhodesia); she lived between her native country and England where she received her education in medicine and psychology. Her first novel, *Nervous Conditions*, was published in 1988 and won the African Section of the Commonwealth Writers Prize. It was followed by a long interruption until the publication of its sequels: *The Book of Not* in 2006 and *This Mournable Body* in 2018. The three novels constitute the Tambudzai and Nyasha trilogy, in reference to the two female protagonists.

Colonialist Conceptions of Nervous Conditions

Dangarembga's trilogy focuses on the intersectional themes of race, gender, and class, from the lenses of Tambu and her cousin Nyasha to examine the pathological consequences of the patriarchal and colonial systems, particularly on females who are burdened with their double oppression. The background is shaped by the sociocultural, historical, political, and economic factors that affected Zimbabwe over the past century. A major historical event that informs the narratives is the colonization of the country, then known as Rhodesia by the British in the 19th century until it gained independence in 1965. The trilogy examines the repercussions of the long-standing colonial rule on the individual and society, including the subjugation of minds, the dispossession of lands, the exploitation of natural resources, and the suppression of local cultures and languages.

The author borrows the title of her first novel in the trilogy, *Nervous Conditions*, from Jean-Paul Sartre's preface to Frantz Fanon's *The Wretched of the Earth* in which he states, "the status of 'native' is a nervous condition introduced and maintained by the colonist in the colonized *with their consent*" (liv). Sartre explains in his preface that colonial power exerts "psychological warfare" on the mind of the colonized to the point of "nervous breakdown" (l); the " 'traumatized,' for life" (li) reacts through violence as an act of cathartic release. These words highlight his existentialist perspective on the relation between colonial domination and psychological manipulation, emphasizing the long-lasting impact on the mental health of the colonized, as well as the consequential expression of violence as a coping mechanism or cathartic response to their psychological struggles.

In the same line of thought, Fanon contends that "violence is a cleansing force" because "It rids the colonized of their inferiority complex, of their passive and despairing attitude" (*The Wretched* 51). He believes that when violence is directed towards each other, particularly against innocent women and children, it is pathological, but when it is directed towards those who have incited it, it is therapeutic. Fanon's provocative views on therapeutic violence are possibly the reason why his vision for psychiatry has not received the attention it merits; his contribution is sometimes obscured by a few pages in which he justifies violent resistance against the inherently violent colonization. In fact, his words on violence are often taken for "a doctrinal prescription" while they can better be considered as a "dramatic dialectical narrative" (Sekyi-Out 4). In other words, Fanon scrutinizes the circumstances that drive to emancipatory violence because for him, "only the armed struggle can effectively exorcize these lies about man that subordinate and literally mutilate the more conscious-minded among us" (*Wretched* 220). Even though he agrees with some colonial psychiatrists that Africans might have violent drives, he refutes the innateness of these drives; he rather attributes them to the oppressive conditions of colonization. For him, therefore, the violence of the colonized is nothing but the natural outcome of the violence of the colonizer, a counter-violence to restore their dignity.

Fanon notes that "the colonized's affectivity is kept on edge like a running sore flinching from a caustic agent. And the psyche retracts, is obliterated, and finds an outlet through muscular spasms that have caused many an expert to classify the colonized as hysterical" (19). For him, the frequent violent confrontations between the colonized and the colonizer induce cumulative psychic wounds that cause a severe erosion of self-esteem. It is not a savage impulse, but a resuscitating action that happens at the very moment when the colonized realize their humanity. The prevalence of violence has left its mark on the colonized against each other; it is a manifestation of the inferiority complex and humiliation that are consuming them, and it hence takes on a cathartic function.

Nervous Conditions: Corporeal Resistance through Eating Disorders

In her trilogy, Dangarembga elaborates on Fanon's work to explore the status of African women oppressed by both the colonial and patriarchal systems. A woman's body speaks for her silenced voice: this is probably the poignant message Dangarembga seeks to transmit on the quest for female identity in an environment of double oppression by patriarchal tradition and colonial education. In the words of Michel Foucault, "nothing is more material, physical, corporal than the exercise of power" (57–58); it "reaches into the very grain of individuals, touches their bodies and inserts itself into their actions and attitudes, their discourses, learning processes and everyday lives" (39). This quote captures the essence of Foucault's theory on power and its pervasive effects on society, penetrating individuals' lives and bodies, disciplining them to conform to societal expectations through various disciplinary institutions and surveillance tools. In an interview with Robtel Neajai Pailey, Dangarembga answers a question on "the psychological manifestations of patriarchy and neo-colonialism on African women and girls (besides eating disorders)." She lists "Low self-esteem; under performance; anti-social behavior; role modeling on anti-social hitherto traditionally masculine behaviors; negative energy; learned helplessness; rage; addiction; alienation; psychological disturbances from neuroses to psychoses; lethargy; dysfunctional attitudes; suicide; self-immolation." This list points up the effects of patriarchal and neo-colonial powers on the mental health of African females. The inclusion of extreme consequences like suicide and self-immolation calls attention to the gravity of the situation and requests an urgent reaction to subvert power relations and build a more equitable society for African women and girls.

Dangarembga's trilogy starts with *Nervous Conditions*, set in colonial Rhodesia in the late 60s to early 70s. Nyasha is the daughter of Babamukuru the patriarch, a school headmaster who studied in England with his wife Maiguru. Their children have spent their early years in England, and when they return to their home country, they suffer from culture shock. They are taught in the missionary school that white men should be treated like deities because they "had come not to take but to give," and that they were animated by performing "God's business" in what they considered as a Dark Continent. The missionaries, the narrator says, "had given up the comfort and security of their homes to come and lighten our darkness. It was a big sacrifice that the missionaries made. It was a sacrifice that made us grateful to them" (105). Dangarembga employs unequivocal irony to critique the "White Man's Burden" or the "Civilizing Mission" ideologies of European imperialism in the 19th century. Rooted in notions of racial and cultural superiority, they were used to justify imperial expansion, claiming that Western powers had a moral obligation to civilize what they called the primitives.

Nyasha cannot understand her parents' changing behaviors and double standards; her father disseminates European egalitarian principles at the mission school, but does not apply them at home. The mother of Tambu, her cousin, describes women's position in her community in these words: "When there are sacrifices to be made, you are the one who has to make them. And these things are not easy; you have to start learning them early [...] and these days it is worse, with the poverty of blackness on one side and the weight of womanhood on the other. Aiwa! What will help you, my child, is to learn to carry your burdens with strength" (16). This piece of advice comes from a woman who toils at home and in the fields without the freedom to voice her grievances; it bears witness to the oppressive nature of patriarchy and the burdens it places on women.

Nyasha, however, refuses these social norms. When her father beats her for behaving like a "whore" and learning to dance with a male friend, she defends herself. Babamukuru is represented as the figure of the colonized man who feels masculine by victimizing colonized women. In his scapegoating mechanism, he channels the violence imposed upon him towards his family. He is the one who suffers from a power-complex caused by his position as a black man in a colonial society, and he reacts by displaying his authority on weaker black females. As Nyasha has no other weapon to fight her oppressor, her resistance to the patriarchal system is corporeal, through eating disorders that metaphorically stand for her endeavor to throw up internal strife. When her father forces her to eat, she defies him by purging herself, reflecting her resistance to his authority. Supriya Nair explains the etiology of her bulimia in the following terms:

> Every instance of bulimic purging comes after a verbal argument with her father, who forces her to eat in order to asset his control. Nyasha's violent purging in the privacy of her bathroom is also indicative of the indigestibility of patriarchal order and discipline, which she nevertheless internalizes in her anorexic condition, the exercise of her will reduces to disciplining and punishing her body. (137)

By forcibly eating and then purging, Nyasha rebels against the indigestible nature of her father's control; her corporeal struggle is a manifestation of her attempt to exercise her will and assert her agency. Her eating disorders are also caused by her inability to reconcile the clashing African and Eurocentric cultures; it is a symptom of being "too Anglicised" (Dangarembga, *Nervous* 74), Tambu's mother observes, "It's the Englishness [...] it will kill them all if they are not careful" (204). The old woman's words reflect the common belief that colonial education, rooted in the imposition of British values, knowledge, and language, disregards the cultural heritage of African societies, disconnecting African youth from their cultural identity and resulting in destructive alienation.

Nyasha has an insatiable appetite for books, which she uses to escape the hysterical climate at home. With each passing moment, however, she discovers the alienating effect of English books, and she frantically tears them up, exclaiming, "We're groveling … for a job … for money. Daddy grovels to them. We grovel to him [...]. Do you see what they've done? They've taken us away [...]. They've deprived you of you, him of him, ourselves of each other [...]. I am not one of them but I'm not one of you" (200–201). This a moment of revelation in which Nyasha understands that books, and the colonial system they represent, have deceived her into believing that she is an educated woman, equal to the white girls with whom she shared the pursuit of knowledge in English schools. Nair considers that Nyasha's action "is also emblematic of the ideological diet of colonial history that literally sickens her [...] Her tearing apart of the colonial textbooks with her teeth, calling them 'bloody lies' suggest her sickness with the ideological diet of colonial history" (137). This powerful act of ripping books with her teeth symbolizes her rebellion against the deceptive and biased narratives imposed on her mind, calling them "bloody lies."

Nyasha is not only bulimic, but also anorexic; she is continually losing weight "from the vital juices she flushed down the toilet" (Dangarembga, *Nervous* 203); she is not aware that her body is becoming "skeletal" and "pathetic" (198), and believes that "angles" are "more attractive than curves" (135). Living in colonial Rhodesia, a country where people suffer from food shortage, her case subverts the country's eating norms, and even the local beauty norms whereby beautiful women should be fleshy. Tambu, who comes from a less privileged family, has a different attitude towards food, "No one who ate from such a table could fail to grow *fat and healthy*" (69, italics added), reflecting the African association between health and fleshiness. Aunt Lucia's "beauty" (125), for instance, is characterized by her plumpness and ability to "cultivate a whole acre single-handed without rest" (127). For this reason, middle-class girls like Nyasha find themselves caught between the simultaneous coexistence of African fat and healthy beauty standards and European slender and sensuous ideals.

Nyasha's anorexia nervosa can be diagnosed as a form of hyper-empathy or "pathological altruism," the tendency of an individual to prioritize other people's requirements above their own in a manner that results in self-damage (Bachner-Melman and Oakley 92). She possesses "an egalitarian nature"; she firmly believes in "the lessons about oppression and discrimination that she had learned firsthand in England" (Dangarembga, *Nervous* 63). She learned about "real peoples and their sufferings" (93) beyond the walls of her affluent family, giving her a sense of guilt over her privileged social position. Her anorexic self-imposed hunger can stand as an act of solidarity with her hungry fellow citizens, an unconscious endeavor to identify with famished Rhodesians. This argument supports her revolt against the colonial system that caused social class disparities, and against her father who represents this system.

Nyasha's mental disorders worsen, and she is admitted to a psychiatric asylum where she requests to be examined by a black psychiatrist. However, as there is no one with this profile, she is examined by a white psychiatrist who believes anorexia nervosa to be quite unlikely in poverty-stricken Rhodesia. Thinking that "Nyasha could not be ill, that Africans did not suffer in the way [they] had described. She was making a scene," he advises her family to "take her home and be firm with her" (206).[20] For the white psychiatrist, therefore, this is a white women's disease, and black women cannot suffer from it unless they are pretending. The attitude of Nyasha's psychiatrist, in Fanon's conception, stems from a deeply ingrained racist ideology that seeks to negate the insidious psychological consequences of oppression, delegitimize resistance, and preserve the dominant colonial order.[21] After her cousin's tragic plight in *Nervous Conditions*, Tambu starts reflecting on her position between two cultures; the novel closes with her words: "It was a long and painful process for me, that process of expansion. It was a process whose events stretched over many years and would fill another volume" (204). The writer is hereby promising a sequel to the novel, actually published no less than 18 years later.

The Book of Not: Corporeal Non-identity

In the second novel in the trilogy, *The Book of Not*, Dangarembga examines the psychological violence experienced by the population during the shift from colonial Rhodesia to independent Zimbabwe, and the focus also shifts from Nyasha to Tambu. In this novel, Nyasha has "missed a year of school" and she has been "partially tranquil by taking plentiful doses of Largactil" (86), to the point of seeming

---

[20] An empirical research on eating disorders among African girls reports only two cases of Zimbabwean upper-class women who studied in England (Brumberg 280).
[21] Fanon explains that such statements, as the one made by Nyasha's psychiatrist, involves a cultural bias that can cause a misdiagnosis. In *Toward the African Revolution*, he considers some mental disorders as pathologies of freedom and vehemently criticizes what colonial psychiatrists called the "North African Syndrome" to describe the fake psychosomatic problems of immigrants. Because this syndrome involves no lesion, they advanced, the immigrants would feign illness to eschew professional obligations, repose in the hospital, and live on the financial assistance of the state (89).

somehow "abject and corpselike" (91). By analogy, psychiatric drugs act like the patriarchal and colonial systems that put her combative mind under control.

This novel opens with a traumatogenic scene in which Tambu witnesses the amputation of her sister Netsai, a guerilla fighter. She feels the straining and tearing of her heart as she views the spinning leg rotating in the air, "Up, up, up, the leg spun. A piece of person, up there in the sky" (3). She sinks into depression and fails to understand her strange seizures and tearful outbursts. She describes her feelings in these words, "It was as if a vital part had been exploded away and in the absence that was left I was cracked and defective, as though indispensable parts leaked, and I could not gather energy" (28). The image of the amputated leg continually haunts Tambu's mind and her violence is symptomatic of a delayed response to trauma. In Dominick LaCapra's theory, when the individual lacks the necessary emotional and cognitive mechanisms to cope with trauma, it can manifest in violent behavior in a desperate effort to externalize negative emotions, stressing the importance of addressing trauma to prevent its transformation into destructive actions. "Acting out" happens when the traumatized is "stuck" in the past, which is natural immediately after the traumatogenic event. Nevertheless, this reaction is pathological if the individual cannot "work through" by using coping healthy strategies like self-examination (148–149). Tambu, however, does not have the coping mechanisms to address her trauma; it leaves her with a persistent numbness that does not recede by the end of the novel, nor in its sequel, *This Mournable Body*.

Tambu is a shortened form of Tambudzai that means "to give trouble" in the local Shona dialect. Her identity is given trouble by the "massive psycho-existential complex" (Fanon, *Black Skin* xvi) that saps her subjectivity. The author draws inspiration from Fanon's example on the child's gaze that "abraded" his body "into nonbeing" (109), causing him to feel "knife blades" within him (118), and perceiving his body as "sprawled out, distorted, recolored, clad in mourning" (113). This example explores the psychological and existential impact of societal forces on an individual, showing that the perception of one's own body can be shaped and distorted by external forces that cause a painful internal experience.

As a black woman, Tambu feels inferior not only to white males and females, but also to black males and younger black females. She feels a sense of shame in the company of her mother, confiding, "in my dealings with Mai, shame welled up. Was there any misfortune in the world as bad as being the daughter of this woman?" (Dangarembga, *The Book* 228). She is also ashamed of her father's poverty and her "unmentionable origin" (231); she finds a sense of pride in joining the house of her uncle (Nyasha's father) for his better social status.

In her effort to reach an important social standing, Tambu becomes fixated on the big Other's recognition ("le grand Autre" in Lacanian terminology)[22]; she toils "to be one of the best," not average, "absolutely outstanding or nothing" (25). In this sense, the title of the novel requests interpellation, as it seems to be a truncated form of *The Book of Not (Being)*. The absence of the word "being" connotes "non-identity"; it also seems to be inspired by Sartre's existentialist reflection on the meaninglessness of life in *Being and Nothingness*[23]. Tambu is the embodiment of the Fanonian "black skin, white masks" syndrome. The "galaxy of erosive stereotypes" (*Black Skin* 129) has resulted in her self-loathing sentiment through the "epidermalization of inferiority" (4). Fanon observes that when the psychic constitution of the black individual is weak, the ego falls apart in contact with the white world. Rather than behaving as an equal human being, the individual behaves in a manner that gratifies the "big Other" to give themselves worth.

Following Lacan's and Fanon's views, Peter Hudson observes that blacks see themselves through the lens of the master signifier of whiteness. In so doing, they perceive themselves, as in a broken mirror, as a distorted "corporeal schema" that provokes a form of mental dismemberment. Believing in "the white order of being with which he seeks to identify," the black subject "sees himself as non-existent" (264), becoming ruptured between two unattainable situations: to be black or white. Being black is "an impossibility in its own terms as there is no black 'being.' " In this non-subject's view, however, being white is made impossible by a segregationist and supremacist system that "is so constructed as to give the black subject nothing to hold onto – no orthopaedic support for an identity," leading to "the ontological void of the black colonized subject" (265). Hudson lays claim to the difficult process of dis-alienation from the pseudo-subject position in the hegemonic order by severing themselves from the "big Other" and "the colonial nothing" that they are (268). It becomes clear, through this analysis, that casting the colonial yoke off the land is easier than casting it off the mind.[24]

The Christian boarding school Tambu attends, called Sacred Heart, claims to be a charitable and equitable institution, but racism is prevalent within its premises. There are spaces, like whites-only toilets, that black girls cannot have access to, and when Tambu is rebuked for using a toilet limited to white girls, she transfers her anger onto her fellow black girls (Dangarembga, *The Book* 71). These black girls are stuffed into a single dormitory; they are frequently insulted by Bougain-

---

[22] See Jacques Lacan's *Le Séminaire livre XVI (1968–1969). D'un Autre à l'autre*. Editions du Seuil, 2006.
[23] See Jean-Paul Sartre's *Being and Nothingness*. Methuen and Company Ltd., 1969.
[24] See Ngũgĩ wa Thiong'o's *Decolonising the Mind: the Politics of Language in African Literature*. Heinemann, 1986.

villea, a white girl who is seldom blamed for her actions. Tambu falls victim to blatant injustice when she achieves the highest score, yet the award goes to the white Tracey for being, allegedly, an "all-rounder" (155). The injustice touches Tambu viscerally, as she feels it "opened up a hole in [her] stomach" (162). The feeling of injustice provokes her psychosomatic symptom, a spasm in the stomach, because of the deep connection between the mind and the body.[25]

Touching between blacks and whites is not allowed in *The Book of Not*, so much so that when Tambu accidentally touches a white teacher's hand, she feels guilty; she reflects, "from the soft warmth upon my skin that Sister and I were in physical contact […] my first impression was I had soiled my teacher in some way. I liked her and I did not want to do that. Sister should not touch me" (31–32). In the same vein, she cannot believe when a black receptionist welcomes her with praise, thinking that "this girl who looked like a goddess was mocking" (214). On the other hand, she considers the disrespectful behavior of the tea boy as normal. It is clear in these numerous instances that Tambu has internalized the "feeling of not existing"; she thinks that "Sin is black as virtue is white" (Fanon, *Black Skin* 106). She feels guilty of some sin, a sin she does not know; colonization has indeed led her to internalize negative stereotypes about the color of her skin.

The traumatic exposure to racial segregation gradually erodes Tambu's sense of self, urging her to delightedly imitate white females and violently treat black ones. Yet, the impossibility of tearing off her black skin and becoming white leads her into a state of not being, hence likely inspiring the choice of the title, *The Book of Not [Being White]*. When, after her graduation, she becomes a teacher at a girls' school, she feels "a smouldering resentment" towards her pupils of the same color. She beats one of them until the victim becomes deaf; she is so shocked by the outcome of her violence that she becomes amnesic and depressive, and she is placed in a mental asylum. As the novel concludes, the homeless and jobless Tambu ruminates: "I had not considered unhu at all, only my own calamities, since the contested days at the convent. So this evening I walked emptily to the room I would soon vacate, wondering what future there was for me, a new Zimbabwean" (246). "Unhu" is the Shona equivalent of "Ubuntu," an African concept that connotes some characteristics like kindness, modesty, empathy, care, respect, responsibility that are apparent in the demeanor, speech, dress, and mainly in the relationship with the family and the society at large (Mandova 357). Had Tambu

---

25 In scientific terms, the stomach is a particularly sensitive area that is influenced by emotions; body stress responses lead to physiological changes including muscle tension and stomach pain.

acted through her trauma with the African philosophy of "Unhu," the author probably means, she would have found a comforting embrace in her community.

Corporeal Grief in *This Mournable Body*

The title of Dangarembga's last novel is probably inspired by two sources. In *Frames of War: When Is Life Grievable?* (2009), Judith Butler maintains, "those whose lives are not 'regarded' as potentially grievable, and hence valuable, are made to bear the burden of starvation, underemployment, legal disenfranchisement, and differential exposure to violence and death" (25). This poignant observation draws attention to the consequences of devaluing certain lives that are not considered worthy of empathy or mourning; it denounces the injustices that result from the differential treatment of lives, and expresses the urgent need for an equal regard for humanity and the worth of all individuals. In *Unmournable Bodies* (2015), Teju Cole equally pays tribute to the victims who "have been killed by U.S. drone strikes in Pakistan and elsewhere" (5), complaining that some victims of violence are given more tribute than others whose lives seem meaningless. He brings awareness to the unequal recognition given to lives lost in acts of violence across the world.

The last novel of Dangarembga's trilogy is about the grief resulting from corporeal hegemony as the author mourns the integrity of the female body at the intersection of patriarchal, colonial, and capitalist systems, calling attention to the urgency of preserving it and giving it due respect. She reflects the feminist view that the female body is reduced to a mere object of male needs, erasing female subjectivity and perpetuating gender inequalities. She vehemently criticizes the patriarchal societies that normalize violence against women's bodies (domestic abuse, sexual assault, or feminicide), perpetuating a culture of silence and blame. Because *This Mournable Body* is a continuation of the reflection started in *Nervous Conditions* and *The Book of Not*, Dangarembga's critique involves the unrealistic beauty standards that fuel body dissatisfaction and self-harm among girls, causing eating disorders like bulimia and anorexia nervosa. She emphasizes that Zimbabwean women's experiences of their bodies, as in other regions of the world, are not only shaped by local cultural norms, but also by global capitalist ones, with conflicting expectations related to leanness and plumpness. By scrutinizing these issues, she probably aims to dismantle the deeply rooted mechanisms that objectify the female body, turning it into a site of resistance and empowerment.

At the beginning of *This Mournable Body*, Tambu is examining the image of her body in the mirror, and she perceives a fish staring back at her; "Its mouth gaping, cheeks dropping as though under the weight of monstrous scales" (18). In this metaphorical description, she engages in self-reflection as the fish-like body image evokes unsettling connotations; it serves as a powerful introduction, setting the stage for the struggle between self-image and societal pressures. The gaping mouth and dropping cheeks evoke her skeletal body and vulnerable mind, recalling the anorexic and pathetic features of her cousin Naysha in *Nervous Conditions*. In *This Mournable Body*, Tambu has not succeeded in making anything of herself; she does not have a job despite her education, and she does not have a communal mooring like her mother, sister, or other women in the village. Without "sustaining family bonds" (37), she cultivates suicidal drives. Nyasha is similarly living in abject poverty despite her education and marriage. It seems that Zimbabwean women, as described by the author, are doomed whatever their educational achievement.

Tambu finds herself in a psychiatric asylum for her physical aggression on a girl who sardonically calls her "Miss Grief." This incident, when examined through a Fanonist lens, shows Tambu's violent response to a system that has perpetuated her perceived inferiority and a manifestation of her anger at being demeaned as "Miss Grief." In her hallucinations, she perceives different sorts of insects like ants and spiders that walk on the walls, reach her bed, and invade her body. She also perceives a scavenging hyena that laughingly intends to devour her corpse. Using the third person pronoun, she says, "She is a corpse, long dead, lying by the bus shelter, dined on by creeping things, gnawed on by scavengers" (205). Her use of the third-person pronoun suggests a dissociation from the experience by considering herself as an external observer, and the hyena reflects her deep-seated vulnerability, a fear of being devoured.

After her psychiatric internment, Tambu lives in extreme destitution at a hostel, facing day-to-day humiliation until Tracey, her former classmate who earlier dispossessed her of her school award in *The Book of Not*, offers her a job in a tourism company. Standing for neoliberal capitalism, Tracey makes a fortune through the commodification of African culture, and Tambu accepts to execute her greedy intentions. Tambu hates going to her village because it reminds her of her "unmentionable origin" (231); she nonetheless returns with a capitalist project that transforms her own mother and other black women into commodities for white tourists by asking them to perform authentic African dances with naked breasts. This commodification reduces local women to objects, stripping them of their agency and dignity; it harks back to a time when colonizers treated Africans as exotic curiosities to be displayed for voyeuristic pleasure. This action can be considered as Tambu's betrayal of her culture, and an expression of her hatred for poor black women; it severs her ties with her community forevermore.

Conclusion

At the end of *Nervous Conditions,* Tambu states, "something in my mind began to assert itself, to question things and to refuse to be brainwashed" (204). This sentence, which shows her determination to benefit from education without losing her own self through it, distressingly, turns into a veneration of white manners in *The Book of Not.* While Nyasha was earlier pacified through tranquilizers, Tambu gradually becomes an alienated and neurotic woman who eventually betrays her own community in *This Mournable Body.* In this light, Dangarembga's education in medicine and psychology, with the influence of Fanon, allowed her to draw a portrait of nervous conditions in postcolonial society, mainly among educated women of tragic fate. She has probed into the body of her society through the minds of her characters to formulate the etiology and diagnosis of her characters' nervous conditions, but she probably has no other restorative therapy to suggest except the traditional "Unhu."

3 Migration Trauma and Presenile Dementia in David Chariandy's *Soucouyant*

Introduction

David Chariandy's *Soucouyant* (2007) explores the themes of migration trauma and presenile dementia from the perspective of a Canadian second-generation immigrant of Caribbean descent. It highlights the way first-generation immigrants can transmit not only their traditions, but also their traumas to their children. Memory, post-memory, and forgetting are essential concepts for the understanding of this novel in which, before forgetting, the protagonist should first go through the difficult phase of remembering. The author voices two generations of immigrants, haunted by the vampiric figure of the "soucouyant," who need to remember their past in order to stay sane in hostile circumstances. He ponders over the meaning of dementia, showing that it eludes precise definitions as it exists beyond what can be fully comprehended or categorized.

Intergenerational Transmission of Migration Trauma

Soucouyant is about Chariandy's first-person experience with intergenerational trauma. The novel is set in Toronto, Ontario, in the late 20th century. Many Caribbeans have migrated to Canada since the 1950s to look for better economic opportunities or to escape sociopolitical unrest in their home countries. The author grew up in the 1970s, during the early years of the government's adoption of the Canadian Multiculturalism Policy (1971). It "was intended to preserve the cultural freedom of all individuals and provide recognition of the cultural contributions of diverse ethnic groups to Canadian society" (*The Canadian Encyclopedia*). Chariandy's novel explores the underlying disparities within Canadian society despite this policy, reflecting the experiences of immigrants and their children who grow up in a racially divided society.

The narrator's mother, Adele, migrated from Trinidad to Toronto in the early 1960s where she frequently encounters racial discrimination. For example, when she wants to buy a lemon meringue pie, the seller asks her to leave the "family restaurant" that does not accommodate "coloureds or prostitutes" (Chariandy, *Soucouyant* 50). She and her husband face challenges in finding an apartment because of their ethnic background, but a property owner reluctantly consents out of monetary necessity (75). The neighbors, however, are outraged by the "intrusion" of colored people in their white neighborhood, so far preserved from the city's "growing ethnic neighborhoods" (59). In the annual "Heritage Day parade," the family are considered as intruders, and publicity flyers differentiate between white Canadians and individuals of "multicultural backgrounds" (60). The discrimination intensifies into racial violence when they return from Niagara Falls to find their home vandalized, with the words "go back" scrawled in excrement on their walls (77). Besides, the narrator's Caribbean accent results in his classification as a "special needs" child (101) and children call him "nigger" at school (157). The hardships endured by the family, including their father's violent death, their son's loss, the narrator's own alienation, and Adele's dementia, seem to be fallouts of deeply ingrained racism.

The family relocates to the less-advantaged Port Junction neighborhood where heavily polluting factories dump chemicals into the local sewage system, resulting in adverse health conditions among the residents. The father suffers from "hacking cough, [...] body stinking of chemicals, [...] heat blisters and funguses" (78). The basement of their house is exposed to toxic substances, including lead and asbestos; the narrator recounts, "I've been feeling tight in my chest and dizzy when standing up too quickly. I lie awake at night in my sleeping bag on my bedroom floor, alternating between nausea and vertigo" (154). In such Toronto neighborhoods, individuals live in insalubrious housing, with problems such as rat and cockroach infestations, unpleasant odors, damaged windows, and insufficient ventilation. This situation becomes an environmental injustice issue due to the presence of a larger proportion of ethnic minorities with low incomes in this neighborhood. The marginalized groups in such areas face disproportionate exposure to health and safety risks caused by hazardous housing. In *Soucouyant*, therefore, the insidious effects of racism and intergenerational trauma intertwine with the cumulative impact of exposure to multiple sources of toxic contamination.

In "When Immigration is Trauma: Guidelines for the Individual and Family Clinician," Rose Marie Perez Foster indicates that migration brings forth numerous emotional and physical challenges, including separation from family, disconnection from the community, and loss of familiar surroundings. Women face particular difficulties due to the absence of established social ties, leading to alienation. Regardless of social or educational background, a decline in socioeconomic status is a common experience for most immigrants, and it can be disheartening for those who hoped for new opportunities in their host country. Perez Foster identifies specific stressors that cause PTSD, anxiety, and depression, associated with the traumatic experiences of immigrants. They are not solely the outcome of migration itself:

1) premigration trauma, i.e., events experienced just prior to migration that were a chief determinant of the relocation; 2) traumatic events experienced during transit to the new country; 3) continuing traumatogenic experiences during the process of asylum-seeking and resettlement; and 4) substandard living conditions in the host country due to unemployment, inadequate supports, and minority persecution. (155)

Perez Foster also points out that a recurring theme in the literature on immigrants' mental health focuses on the psychological response of mothers to stressors before migration because it can serve as an indicator of the mental well-being of their children (158).

To represent his mother's trauma, the author borrows the motif of the "soucouyant" that represents not only the hardships she has endured because of racism in Canada but also the deep-seated wounds stemming from her childhood experiences in Trinidad. The "soucouyant" is a female vampire in Caribbean mythology who, during the day, lives in the skin of a sequestered old woman, and during the night, tears her skin and metamorphoses into a wandering fireball. Her victims are pale and bear a "telltale mark or bruise"; the narrator explains,

> A soucouyant is something like a female vampire. She lives a reclusive but fairly ordinary life on the edge of town. She disguises herself by dressing up in the skin of an old woman, but at night she'll shed her disguise and travel across the sky as a ball of fire. She'll hunt out a victim and suck his blood as he sleeps, leaving him with little sign of her work except increasing fatigue, a certain paleness, and perhaps, if he were to look closely on his body, a tell-tale bruise or mark on his skin. (Chariandy, *Soucouyant* 135)

The gothic use of this vampiric creature unites the thematic threads of the novel and serves as a tool to articulate the narrative of migration trauma and presenile dementia. The gothic genre, with its themes of madness, the uncanny, and the supernatural, provides a rich symbolic framework that represents the haunting and unsettling experiences of individuals affected by traumatic conditions. It embodies notions of loss, displacement, and the devouring of one's sense of self (Edwards 50). By employing gothic imagery, Chariandy can capture the psychological and emotional dimensions of migration trauma and presenile dementia, giving shape to the feelings of anxiety and alienation that often accompany the victims. In addition, the gothic narrative allows for a symbolic exploration of the power dynamics and sense of otherness experienced by immigrants in their new environments where they may be perceived as monstrous.

Adele needs not only to face the hardship of integration into the host country, but also to forget her pre-migration trauma. Her problem started in her childhood; to afford the family's living, her mother was a prostitute during the American Occupation of Trinidad in the 1940s. The young Adele was seduced to become a prostitute, at the age of seven, by an American soldier who gave her presents "from afar," including pictures of Hollywood stars, chewing gum, and chocolate, tokens of the neocolonial expansionism[26] that started at that time (Chariandy, *Soucouyant* 188). Despite her efforts to suppress the memory, the traumatic image of her mother is constantly resurfacing as she remembers her "in a dress of fire' (193). This story, transmitted in fragments by Adele to her son, indicates that she "forget[s] to forget" (32), meaning that she is forgetting many aspects of everyday life, but not this traumatic event that happened in the distant past. Susan J. Brison explains that traumatic memories "are experienced by the survivor as inflicted, not chosen"; they are usually "uncontrollable, intrusive" (40). The burden of memory can be relieved by talking to what Brison calls a "second person" who can piece together the fragmented narrative. This "second person" for Adele is her son who attempts to piece together her life story. He cares for his mother in her advanced state of dementia, trying to piece together her life story, starting in Trinidad, her displacement during the war, her migration to Canada, and finally her illness and death. He attempts to reconstruct them into narrative, structured like a tale, beginning with "there was once a girl named Adele" (Chariandy, *Soucouyant* 180), as if the mother is a person other than the listener.

In an interview with Kit Dobson, Chariandy expresses his wish to provide a fresh perspective on memory loss. He affirms, "I'm indeed dabbling with casting forgetting in more creative and at least not-wholly-pejorative terms – a desire motivated both by my sympathies towards people with dementia, and a critical take on what you might call nostalgic or naïve recuperative agendas" ("Spirits" 813). In the novel, therefore, the son discovers that his mother's memories are buried inside his "sleeping self"; he mumbles the word "soucouyant" in his sleep (Chariandy, *Soucouyant* 32), implying that the mother's trauma has been transmitted to him.

Because the son cannot complete the story on his own, he asks his mother about the way her burns were treated; she answers, "'Oh dear,' [...] Whatever you think you want with some old nigger-story?'" (194). Failing to find an answer in his mother's words, Chariandy tries to provide one in an interview with Kate Kellawey; he contends, "The past is not yet past. When things happen, the only way we can make sense of it is by telling the story about the past – realising where prejudices come from. And the point would be not only to spin a story about racial violence but to tell how our ancestors have bravely and creatively

---

[26] This period was marked by neocolonial imperialism, during which colonial powers exploited less powerful countries for their own advantage. Given Trinidad's oil and bauxite resources, the island was subject to various forms of environmental and human exploitation (Chariandy, *Soucouyant* 177–178).

overcome these things." He acknowledges the enduring influence of the past on the present and emphasizes the necessity of comprehending the way it shapes racial prejudice. Importantly, his later novel, *I've Been Meaning to Tell You: A Letter to my Daughter* (2018) is a testament to his desire to break the cycle of intergenerational trauma. He tells his 13-year-old daughter, "Now you speak your own truths and you will continue to find the scripts that honour your body and experience and history, each of these scripts a gift, and none of them fully adequate to the holy force of you" (84). With heartfelt determination to safeguard his daughter's mental well-being in a world tainted by racial prejudice, the father's uplifting words resonate powerfully: "You are not what they see and say you are. You are more" (120). He obviously wants to relieve his daughter from the burden of memory, intergenerational migration trauma, and other mental disorders with which he and his mother have been struggling.

Presenile Dementia as a Compounding Factor for Migration Trauma

In *Soucouyant*, Chariandy uses presenile dementia as a compounding factor that aggravates the migration trauma and racial injustice to which Adele is subject. Presenile dementia is a neurological disease characterized by progressive deterioration of cognitive abilities; it leads to impairment in daily functioning, mood swings, memory loss, and communication difficulties. When the son returns to his mother after an absence of two years, she has become a completely different woman who screams when touched, destroys kitchen tools while trying to cook, and even confuses her son with her dead husband. In a state of disorientation, her condition leads her to roam the neighborhood partially naked, uttering incoherent expressions, and engaging in uncommon behaviors such as urinating in inappropriate places.

The narrator believes the dementia of his mother finds its roots in the traumatic fire she survived during her childhood in Trinidad, as she is constantly haunted by the memory of this fire and the related fireball-like mythical vampire. He depicts the heavy effects of the disease on the patients' memory, as well as the emotional toll it takes on them and their families:

> During our lives, we struggle to forget. And it's foolish to assume that forgetting is altogether a bad thing. Memory is a bruise still tender. History is a rusted pile of blades and manacles. And forgetting can sometimes be the most creative and life-sustaining thing that we can ever hope to accomplish. The problem happens when we become too good at forgetting. When somehow we forget to forget, and we blunder into circumstances that we consciously should have avoided. This is how we awaken to the stories buried deep within our sleeping selves. (32)

In this philosophical passage on the ebb and flow of memory caused by dementia, forgetting takes on a subtle meaning. As individuals review the trajectory of their lives, they try to find a delicate balance between remembering and forgetting. The act of forgetting is not necessarily disadvantageous, as it can be a protective mechanism to soothe the wounds of memory. The accumulation of experiences leaves behind marks like bruises from a history fraught with suffering. In some instances, forgetting becomes a powerful tool that allows individuals to go through the challenges of life, but it becomes perilous when it lets go of essential memories and life lessons that need to be cherished.

The Canadian doctor finds it difficult to establish Adele's diagnosis because he does not grasp "the many unusual features of Mother's case." He is disoriented about how "early the symptoms had appeared and how slowly and unevenly they had developed" (37). He says, "Although the SWR or Standard Word Recall test, may offer preliminary indications of the condition [dementia], one must be cautious. Depression and certain post-traumatic states may produce false positives. One must especially be cautious when dealing with the uneducated and/or ethnic minorities" (41). In the case of false positives, the doctor argues, the SWR test indicates the presence of dementia when, in reality, the individual does not have the condition. It means that other factors, such as depression or post-traumatic disorders, may be influencing the test outcome. This is particularly possible when the test is administered to individuals who may have limited education or belong to ethnic minorities. This might be true because Adele has often been "suspicious about medical institutions and offices" (39), and she would be reluctant to disclose her full being. In the context of migration, as Foster affirms, individuals may experience a sense of shame when sharing their experiences of vulnerability with a clinician who is ethnically unfamiliar (155). There is probably an unconscious inclination to repress memories of highly distressing and ego-disrupting events.

By the end of the novel, Adele falls down the stairs and hits her head. Her son finds "a spot of blood" on her forehead as if marked by the bite of the "soucouyant" (Chariandy, *Soucouyant* 138). After her death, he discovers a "telltale mark or bruise" (135) on his forehead too, symbolizing the intergenerational trauma from which he is unable to escape despite his Canadian birth. The son's inheritance of his mother's "soucouyant" bruise recalls what Marianna Hirsch calls "postmemory," a valuable theoretical lens through which to examine the intergenerational dynamics of memory processes, particularly in the transmission of traumatic memories. She says,

> "Postmemory" describes the relationship that the "generation after" bears to the personal, collective, and cultural trauma of those who came before-to experiences they "remember" only by means of the stories, images, and behaviors among which they grew up. But these

experiences were transmitted to them so deeply and affectively as to seem to constitute memories in their own right. [...] To grow up with overwhelming inherited memories, to be dominated by narratives that preceded one's birth or one's consciousness, is to risk having one's own life stories displaced, even evacuated, by our ancestors. (106–107)

This explains the relationship that the "generation after" a traumatic event has with the experiences and memories of those who came before them. It suggests that the "generation after" only has access to these experiences through the stories, images, and behaviors that shaped their upbringing. Despite not experiencing these events in a direct manner, they are deeply and effectively transmitted to them, leading to a sense of these experiences becoming their own memories. Hirsch points out the potential for personal narratives to be eclipsed by the overwhelming presence of parental memories.

Clearly, as Adele's memories of her history in Trinidad fade away, her son becomes burdened with the weight of remembering that history. Chariandy explains that Adele's dementia "enabled [him] to explore the fragility and endurance of cultural memory, and, most particularly, the challenge of cultural memory for a second-generation migrant" ("Spirits" 813). In this quote, he elucidates that Adele's dementia allows him to explore the relationship between vulnerability and resilience. He also shows the difficulties he has been facing as a second-generation immigrant, as well as the responsibility of preserving the weight of memory that falls upon him.

Conclusion

In Chariandy's *Soucouyant*, migration trauma and presenile dementia unfold through the eyes of a second-generation Canadian of Caribbean heritage. In a process of "rememory," the narrative traces the transmission of trauma between generations as the protagonist embarks on a challenging journey of remembrance before ultimately facing the value of forgetting. The two generations of immigrants struggle with the haunting presence of the "soucouyant," the Caribbean fireball vampire, as they constantly remember their tormented past. Contemplating the meaning of dementia, the narrator realizes that it defies precise definition, but he learns the importance of forgetting the dark facets of his story/history in order to maintain his sanity. In so doing, the author reveals his intention to provide a fresh outlook on memory loss, combining empathy for those suffering from dementia and critical examination of overly nostalgic attempts to reclaim the past.

Part IV: **Disability in the Global Anglophone Novel**

1 Beyond "Narrative Prosthesis": Disability Interpretations in Bapsi Sidhwa's *Cracking India*

Introduction

Bapsi Sidhwa's *Cracking India: A Novel* (1991), previously published as *Ice Candy Man* (1988), is a historical narrative in which the devastating polio disease may be interpreted as a symbol of colonialism while the cracking of plaster might be a metaphorical representation of Indian Partition. The author is a highly acclaimed Pakistani writer born in 1938, seven years before the Partition of India that she witnessed with the eyes of a child. Most plausibly, her protagonist stands for Pakistan, the youthful and scarred nation that arose from the Partition of India in 1947, confirming Mitchell and Snyder's view that disability usually serves as a metaphoric "clutch" or "narrative prosthesis" (49) in this novel to stand for colonial violence and corporeal agency. It is, however, an under-interpretation to stop at this discursive level because, using Quayson's typology of disability representation, the novel can be placed under the third category, "*Disability as articulation of disjuncture between thematic and narrative vectors*" (41). It is likewise useful to read it in terms of the ninth category, "*Disability as normality*" (52) because the protagonist seems to be content with her disability, in a manner that corroborates the social model of disability.

Game Plan of "Divide and Rule"

Sidhwa's *Cracking India: A Novel* reflects on the historical events and social issues that shaped the lives of millions of people during the British colonial decision to leave the Indian subcontinent. The Partition resulted in widespread displacement (see figure 11) and violence between Hindu, Muslim, and Sikh communities, with estimates of one million casualties and fourteen to eighteen million refugees (Dyson 189). The novel reflects, in addition to the trauma of loss and dismemberment, on the issues of religion, class, and gender. It illustrates the bloody conflicts between religious communities that are exploited by political leaders, as it features female characters who struggle against the patriarchal norms of their society.

In *Cracking India: A Novel*, Sidhwa seems to make a claim that British rulers bear responsibility for the tragic consequences of the Partition, as they hastily decided to divide India into two countries before their withdrawal. The inadequately planned decision has resulted in a catastrophic situation comparable to the perma-

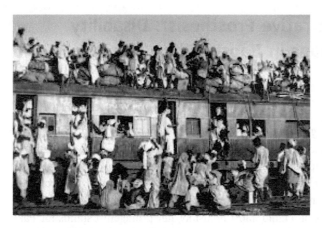

Figure 11: A Station Near Delhi (Partition of India, 1947) (Public domain image, reproduced from Columbia Mealac Pritchett Routes Data. www.columbia.edu/itc/mealac/pritchett/00routesdata/1900_1999/partition/trains/trains.html

nent disfigurement caused by polio in Lenny's leg. Colonel Bharucha, her doctor, blames the British for her contracting polio, drawing a parallel between the damaging effects of the virus and the historical alterations imposed by the British on the subcontinent. He says, "If anyone's to blame, blame the British! There was no polio in India till they brought it here!" (16). Lenny is the child narrator of the novel who, with the mind of an adult, reflects, "'The goddamn English!' [...] 'They gave us polio!' And notwithstanding the compatible and sanguine nature of my relationship with my disease, I feel it is my first personal involvement with Indian politics" (26). This quote indicates that even if Lenny has come to accept her disability, she condemns the British for transmitting it to her countrymen who do not all have the same privileged position to cope with it. She further explains the role of polio in her political involvement in the "Quit-India sentiment," as she takes part, despite her young age, in the widespread anti-colonial movement to end the British Raj.

Many Indians and Pakistanis hold the British responsible for the long-lasting strife between the different religious communities through the creation of socioeconomic inequality and political rivalry. Indian jurist Justice Markandey Katju recounts that in the anti-colonial revolt known as the "Great Mutiny" (1857), Hindus and Muslims joined forces in their resistance against British colonial rule. This event unsettled the British government and incited it to adopt the political strategy of "divide and rule" to quell the Mutiny and avoid the recurrence of similar revolts. Katju argues that the ensuing communal riots were "artificially engineered by the British authorities." In their covert scheme, they would clandestinely provide financial incentives to Hindu Pandits, instructing them to propagate anti-Muslim sentiments. Similarly, they would offer monetary inducements to Muslim Maulvis, encouraging them to express hostility towards Hindus (7). This deliberate injection of communal animosity became a characteristic of the Indian political landscape.

Literary Representations of Disability

Due to contracting polio at a young age, Sidhwa had undergone surgery and received home tutoring until she turned fifteen. In the novel, therefore, she overlaps the two traumatic narratives that shaped her childhood. She juxtaposes the experiences of Lenny, the four-year-old protagonist who contracts polio and undergoes surgery with the traumatic history of Partition. In his typology of disability representation, Quayson classifies Sidhwa's *Cracking India* under the third category, "*Disability as articulation of disjuncture between thematic and narrative vectors*" (41), in which the character with disability, Lenny, lies at the center of the dissociation between content and form. She unrealistically acts like an adult when she addresses the reader, but she remains a child in her interactions with the other characters of the novel.

The title is constructed on the allegory of cracking Lenny's plaster and her attempt to walk without limping, in relation to the cracking of India through Partition. Lenny says, "I stare at the white plaster forcing my unique foot into the banal mold of a billion other feet and I ponder my uncertain future" (Sidhwa 18). The emaciated and wrinkled leg stands for Pakistan, the "toddler nation greenly fluttering its flag" (286), for which the novel has been criticized as perpetuating the colonial stereotype of the nation as a child. "The disabled child-nation trope," Clare Barker argues, "has its antecedents in a long colonial history in which childhood and disability contributed substantially to the conceptual apparatus of empire" (7). This representation stresses the power dynamics inherent in colonialism where dependency and vulnerability are associated with disability and childhood.

One of the most pivotal moments in the novel is one in which Lenny's emotional distress compels her to dismember her "bloated celluloid doll" (Sidhwa 138). By replicating the witnessed violence and mutilating the inanimate object, she manifests the chaos within her psyche. In the midst of unimaginable violence, by good fortune, the presence of the loving figure of the grandmother brings solace to Lenny. She says, "Godmother sits by my bed smiling indulgently while men in uniforms quietly slice off a child's arm here, a leg there. She strokes my head as they dismember me. I feel no pain. Only an abysmal sense of loss-and a chilling horror that no one is concerned by what's happening" (22). This is a testament to the enduring power of love, even in the face of unspeakable trauma.

Sidhwa, who belongs to the Parsi community, uses a Parsi narrator to provide a somewhat neutral perspective to her portrayal of communal violence. Lenny spends most of her time with Ayah Shanta, the Hindu nanny, and Imamdin, the Muslim cook, demonstrating the existence of communal harmony prior to the Partition. The adult-child lies at the center of the fragmented narrative of *Cracking India* and serves as a reflection of the shattered state of both the nation and the individual following the Partition. Just as the Partition cleaved the Indian subcontinent into two nations, the narrative structure is characterized by fragmentation, with vivid descriptions of physical crumbling, tearing, cracking, bleeding, and suffering. The frequent references to bodily fragmentation also symbolize the rupturing of personal identities, as characters are torn apart from their roots, homes, and loved ones.

It is also possible to reflect on *"Disability as normality"* (Quayson 52) in this novel because Lenny seems to be a normal human being with a full range of emotions, contradictions, aspirations, and worries; she seems to be a self-satisfied, even captivating, character. She mainly "cultivates her limp as her marker of privilege" (Barker 104). She demonstrates self-awareness regarding her vulnerability as a child affected by polio, as she skillfully influences the adults to obtain information. She is also a privileged child with a disability because she grows up in a loving and affluent family. Her disability elicits feelings of guilt in her mother who thinks she neglected her by leaving her in the care of a nanny; she usually massages her daughter's leg and diverts her attention from her pain by telling stories and playing tricks. The socioeconomic status of Lenny's family affords her the advantage of receiving education from a private tutor, but it hinders her ability to interact with other children in an inclusive environment.

When Lenny goes for a walk with her nanny, she notices her difference through the other's gaze; she observes, "I observe the curious glances coming my way and soak in the commiserate clucking of tongues, wearing a polite and nonchalant countenance. [...] despite the provocative agitation of Ayah's bouncy walk, despite the gravitational pull of her moon-like face, I am the star attraction of the street" (Sidhwa 9). In this other's gaze, however, there is no apparent stigmatization, but empathy and benevolence. Interestingly, the gaze empowers Lenny as she openly expresses her appreciation of her condition. She wonders, "Will I have to behave like other children, slogging for my share of love and other handouts?" Considering the advantages of having a disability, she adds, "Having polio in infancy is like being born under a lucky star. It has many advantages – it permits me to access to my mother's bed in the middle of the night" (10). Having gained this much love and attention from her family and household workers, she worries that the surgery would correct her leg, suppress her identity as a polio-affected girl, and let her resemble "other" girls. In this figurative dimension, Lenny embraces her physical weakness as a symbol of her privileged status, a "valuable deformity" (15). Despite her young age, Lenny subverts the "history of assigned corporeal inferiority so that bodily differences become markers of exceptionality to be claimed and honored" (Garland-Thomson 18). Her case illustrates the social model of disability, highlighting the role society plays in worsening the experience of impaired corporeality.

Lenny's contentment with her disability serves as a confirmation that the true burden lies not in the physical impairment itself, but rather in the societal response it engenders. The novel, written in the 1980s when various disability rights groups were actively shaping the discourse around disability, subtly reflects the emergence of the social model of disability, a concept coined by Mike Oliver.[27] In this model, disability is not solely a result of an individual's physical or mental impairment, but also the product of societal barriers and attitudes towards this individual. Lenny's case is an illustration of how an individual with a disability can lead a normal life when surrounded by loving affection.

Bharat Mata: **The Embodiment of Motherhood and Victimhood**

The Partition of India caused immense suffering for women who were the primary victims of its brutalities; they were abducted and raped while their children were killed on both sides of the border. In line with the patriarchal reasoning that led to the widespread sexual assault on women belonging to another religious group, there were instances of women who resorted to suicide or were subject to homicide by male relatives. The following passage unveils the macabre scene of a train arriving from Gurdaspur where a massacre left no survivors; "everyone in it is dead butchered. There are no young women among the dead! Only two young gunny bags full of women's breasts" (Sidhwa 159). This is a poignant example of extreme human cruelty. The absence of young women among the victims suggests their exploitation as either servants or prostitutes while the presence of breasts serves as a reminder that the female body is often the locus of mutilation.

The pain of Partition is compared to the pain of childbirth. People say, "We've given birth to a new nation. Pakistan!" (151). By equating the Indian nation with the woman's body of *"Bharat Mata"* (Mother India, see figure 12) and Pakistan with childhood dependency, the narrative reinforces the nationalist idea of Indian superiority. Likewise, Ayah, the attractive Hindu woman, may represent Mother India whose sensual physicality contrasts with the aging body of Mrs. Pen, the Eng-

---

27 See Mike Oliver's *Social Work with Disabled People*. Macmillan, 1983.

lish woman. Ayah's seductive presence also challenges the authority of the imposing statue of Queen Victoria in the park, and her allure reflects anti-colonial sentiment and Indian nationalism. As her love affair with a Muslim character unfolds, Ayah symbolizes a potential alliance between Hindus and Muslims within the envisioned nation. After the violent Partition, however, a question arises concerning her beauty and vitality: "Where have the radiance and the animation gone? Can the soul be extracted from its living body?" (272). Interpreting the quote as Ayah standing for India, it conveys the sense of loss and despair induced by the Partition upon the nation.

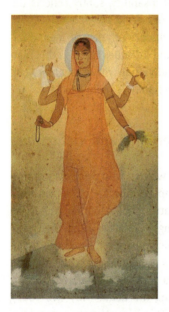

Figure 12: Abanindranath Tagore's "Bharat Mata" (1905, public domain image) www.partitionstudiesquarterly.org/article/1905-cartography-nationalism-and-iconography/

Eventually, Lenny realizes that the prevalence of violence in her community is largely influenced by gender. As violence escalates, Ayah is abducted by Ice Candy Man, a nationalist leader engaged in political and religious rhetoric. In response to this traumatic event, Lenny experiences distress and exhibits bulimic symptoms. For three days, she would face the bathroom mirror, grasp the "truth-laden" organ (tongue) between her fingers, attempting to discipline it with an abrasive toothbrush until it painfully bleeds (Sidhwa 184). The vivid imagery conveys Lenny's desire to rid herself of the truth that infects her being.

Conclusion

Sidhwa's *Cracking India* weaves together the historical narrative of the Indian Partition and the personal narrative of disability. Through the polio disease, she illustrates the lasting impact of colonialism on the nation, and the metaphorical representation of the cracking plaster is a reminder of the shattered lives and traumatic grief caused by the Partition. Lenny's embodiment of Pakistan, emerging as a young but wounded nation, aligns with Mitchell and Snyder's notion that disability often functions as a metaphorical "clutch" for colonial violence. However, it would be an incomplete interpretation to consider disability only through this lens. By examining Quayson's typology of disability representation, the novel falls into the categories of *"Disability as articulation of disjuncture between thematic and narrative vectors"* (41) and *"Disability as normality"* (52). As the character with a disability appears content with her condition, the novel calls attention to the social model of disability and the role of benevolence in alleviating the pain of the disability experience.

2 Ableism and Disgrace in Salman Rushdie's *Shame*

Introduction

Salman Rushdie's *Shame* (1983) is an allegorical representation of disability in the context of Pakistani sociopolitical history. It can be interpreted through the lens of "narrative prosthesis" (Mitchell and Snyder 49) due to its heavily metaphorical use of disability. The main character, seemingly suffering from an autistic disorder, is portrayed in ableist terms as a bestial being. The chapter draws upon the medical, social, and moral models of disability to offer a more empathic interpretation, examining the character through a more humane lens. It also provides alternative interpretations through Quayson's fourth type of disability representation, *"Disability as bearer of moral deficit/evil"* (42) as well as the seventh type, *"Disability as inarticulable and enigmatic tragic insight"* (49).

Disability Models and Ableist Stereotypes

The understanding of disability encompasses various models that offer distinct perspectives on its nature and implications. The moral model, which has persisted throughout history, frames disability within a moral or religious context, associating it with divine punishment. Proponents of this model perceive disability as "a defect caused by moral lapse or sins" (Olkin 25). Traces of this model persist, such as in popular culture, in which individuals with disabilities are frequently depicted as antagonists or malevolent figures. The beginning of the medical model can be traced back to the 19th century, a period marked by significant scientific advancements that enhanced the comprehension of disabilities and their causes. It views disability as "a defect in or failure of a bodily system and as such is inherently abnormal and pathological" (26). In contrast, the social model, which started in the 20th century, redirects attention from the individual's impairment to the societal obstacles that impede complete participation and inclusion. Impairment is defined as a "limitation in a person's physical, mental or sensory functioning" which becomes "salient and disabling in specific settings" (Marks 80). Proponents of this model perceive disability as existing within the social environment, which they see as exclusionary and oppressive, rather than inherent in the body.

Ableism refers to discrimination against persons with disabilities, treating them as inferior and denying them equal opportunities based on the belief that able-bodiedness is the norm. It manifests on both institutional and interpersonal levels; institutional forms include social barriers within societal structures that sustain discrimination while interpersonal manifestations involve repressive attitudes and interactions. These two levels can lead to disability becoming internalized through self-stigmatization (Campbell 20). From another angle, ableism is lived in different forms, "from the seemingly benevolent to the blatantly hostile, and more ambivalent or mixed forms" (Nario-Redmond et al. 726). In Rushdie's *Shame*, ableism seems to be institutional, interpersonal, and "blatantly hostile" toward Sufiya Zinobia, the character with a disability, including countless examples of overt discrimination and explicit humiliation. Throughout the novel, if she is not presented as a simpleton, she is presented as a demon. In the figure of the simpleton, mortifying terms towards her abound, like "damaged child," "deranged daughter," "simpleton girl," "stunted intelligence," and "broken mind." The following are further instances in which she is described in the most humiliating terms:

- "A simpleton, a goof!" (101)
- "Straw instead of cabbage between the ears. Empty in the breadbin. To be done? But darling, there is nothing. That birdbrain, that mouse! I must accept it: she is my shame [the mother is speaking]" (101).
- "The idiot child whose mother called her 'shame' and treated her like mud" (119).
- "Sufiya Zinobia, the idiot, is blushing" (120).
- The "deranged daughter," at the age of "twenty-eight had advanced to a mental age of approximately nine and a half" (218).

In the representation of Sufiya as a "somnolent demon," she sleepwalks and beheads two hundred and eighteen turkeys, tearing "off their heads" and reaching down "into their bodies to draw their guts up through their necks with her tiny weaponless hands" (138). Her decapitation reaches humans when she threatens to kill the bridegroom during her sister Naveed's wedding ceremony; she buries her teeth in his neck, and when he escapes her bite, she keeps "a morsel of his skin and flesh in her teeth" (171). Eventually, without her consent, she enters into an arranged marriage with Omar Khayyam Shakil who needs a strategic alliance with her influential father. The husband, a doctor, keeps her sedated and savors his time with her servant. When Sufiya, whose matrimonial rights are unfulfilled, discovers the adultery, she becomes bestial; "she was there, on all fours, naked, coated in mud and blood and shiny, with twigs sticking to her back and beetles in her hair"; Omar "stood before her, unable to move, her hands, her wife's hands, reached out to him and closed" (286). The imagery of Sufiya on all fours, naked, and covered in mud and blood suggests a loss of humanity and a descent into a more animalistic state.

In the previous example, Sufiya goes wild because her marital rights are withheld due to stereotypical assumptions that infantilize and asexualize her. In *The Sexual Politics of Disability: Untold Desires*, Tom Shakespeare et al. explore the relationship between disability and sexuality. According to the authors, disabled men, and to a lesser extent women, are often perceived as impotent and devoid of sexual desire due to their disabilities; they are considered unattractive and susceptible to ridicule. This perception of sexual inadequacy can lead to the involvement in extramarital relationships. This phenomenon is referred to as the "Chatterley Syndrome" after D.H. Lawrence's *Lady Chatterley's Lover* in which the eponymous character seeks sexual fulfillment with a "manly man" because her husband is physically disabled. Persons with disabilities, Shakespeare et al. add, are often represented as either devoid of any sexual agency, as asexual beings or as perversely hypersexualized (87). This is the picture the novel provides of Sufiya who, in one scene, partakes in physical intimacy with four adolescents before decapitating them.

Rushdie presents Sufiya as the misshapen villain who represents "*Disability as bearer of moral deficit/evil*" (Quayson 42), illustrating the moral model of disability which views it as an individual's moral flaw, a punishment or a consequence of their actions. This model often leads to stigmatization and shame, as the individual with a disability is considered morally inferior. The shame extends to the whole family that considers the birth of a child with a disability as a curse. In Rushdie's novel, Sufiya is the victim of the (m)other's gaze, right from the cradle; her mother laments that her husband "wanted a hero of a son"; she "gave him an idiot instead," and she considers her "the incarnation of their shame" (210). Consequently, "The plague of shame spread rapidly through that tragic being [Sufiya] whose chief defining characteristic was her sensitivity to the bacilli of humiliation" (141), and she grows up with an uncontrollable tendency to blush whenever she faces other people's gaze.

As the previous passages illustrate, persons with disabilities often encounter a deficiency in affection that is necessary for their emotional growth. Rather than receiving love and warmth at home, they are subjected to abuse and condemnation. The parents in Rushdie's novel have two daughters, one of whom, Sufiya, nicknamed Shame, and the other, Naveed, nicknamed Good News. This naming practice substantiates the role of parental attitudes in the victimization experienced by children with disabilities at the hands of their family. Bilquis, the mother, lavishes all her affection on her other daughter, Naveed, while Sufiya is burdened by her mother's sense of shame and remains emotionally barren. The narrator recounts, "Groans, insults, even the wild blows of exasperation rained on her instead; but such rain yields no moisture. Her spirit parched for lack of affection, but she nevertheless managed, when love was in her vicinity, to glow happily just to be near the precious thing" (121). She internalizes the language of shame from her early interactions with her parents and significant others who direct a continuous stream of shaming words and actions, leading her to feel defective.

Sufiya's mental disorder is not clearly diagnosed, but the etiology is attributed to three possible causes: the girl "contracted a case of brain fever that turned her into an idiot" (100); she is a punishment for her mother's sins (101), or her brain has been damaged by the "continuous blows her mother rained on her head" (109). From a medical viewpoint, however, her symptoms might indicate that she has an Autism Spectrum Disorder (ASD), identified by "the core features of social communication issues and the presence of restricted and/or repetitive behaviours that variably but significantly impact on quality of life" (Whiteley 1). Sufiya usually tears "each damaged hair in two, all the way down to the roots" (Rushdie 136). Her vacant eyes, averted gaze, penchant for rearranging furniture and caressing pebbles are indicative of autism symptoms. Furthermore, the narrator indicates that her "body's defence mechanism has declared war against the very life they are supposed to be protecting" (142). The reference to brain fever and body's defense mechanism waging war against itself indicates that Sufiya's diagnosis might be Autoimmune Encephalitis (AE). The disease is characterized by the immune system's attack on normal brain cells, causing inflammation, fever, as well as cognitive and psychiatric manifestations that are similar to Autism Spectrum Disorders (Whiteley 1). What is striking in the existing medical literature is that extreme violence is not a defining characteristic of autism (Rutten 8). In this case, Sufiya's aggressive behavior quite possibly stems from social stigma and the resulting communication disorder, emotional conflict, and internalized ableism.

Intersections of "Narrative Prosthesis" and "Aesthetic Nervousness"

Rushdie's *Shame* is the illustration of Mitchell and Snyder "narrative prosthesis" par excellence because it employs disability as a "crutch" the narrative leans on "for the representational power, disruptive potentiality, and analytical insight" (49). The Novel is an allegory of Pakistan during the reign of Muhammad Zia-ul-Haq (1978–1988), a period marked by authoritarian rule and corruption. He is represented by General Raza Hyder, Sufiya's father, and the country is named "Peccavistan," the nation that is, like Sufiya, "a miracle that went wrong" (86). The novel revisits the historical power struggle in Pakistan between General Zia Ul-Haq and Zulfikar Ali Bhutto. Omar Khayyam Shakil is the figure of the Westernized and shameless opportunist. He marries the shame-ridden Sufya to get a privileged position in her father's entourage, "attempting a shameless piece of social climbing [...] by marrying the unmarriageable child" (156). Both the father and the husband are notorious for their subservient loyalty to foreign powers and their policies of interference, causing hostility among the populace.

In reality, General Zia Ul-Haq had a daughter with a disability, called Zian, who served as an inspiration for Sufiya. She is represented in the novel as the "disorder's avatar" (Rushdie 200), and her disability serves as a "prosthesis" that propels the storyline forward. She embodies the prevalent corruption inherent in the political sphere, and her ability to metamorphose can be a metaphorical representation of the alluring aspects of power, capable of captivating and exerting influence over individuals. Her father and her husband involve her in political maneuvers as a strategic instrument to consolidate their power. Considering this portrayal of Zian Zia Ul-Haq through the character of Sufiya, the reader is compelled to contemplate the indignation and mortification that would inevitably befall her guiltless person in reality.

Another interpretation might be, beyond the surface level, that the author is deliberately presenting the character with a disability in a shocking and derogatory manner to provoke a response from the readers and raise awareness about their own ableism. In this sense, Quayson's concept of "aesthetic nervousness" can be detected in the connection between the text and the readers who observe the difficulties faced by a character with a disability in an ableist society (15). Hence, readers are challenged to "lift [their] eyes from the reading of literature to attend more closely to the implications of the social universe around [them]" (31). In reading Rushdie's *Shame*, they are prompted to critically examine the portrayal of Sufiya, stripped of her personhood, womanhood, and motherhood. Approaching the character with empathy, despite her described metaphorical bestiality, readers can observe Sufiya from an endearing angle. In some instances, she plays with babies; "The best thing that has happened recently is the babies, her sisters' babies. She, Sufiya, plays with them as often as she can" (273). Ableists tell her, cruelly, "babies aren't for you" (236). Because no love or attention is directed towards her, she caresses pebbles, and she radiates with delight when she hears words of affection albeit addressed to other persons.

In light of this, Sufiya's case fully illustrates the view that reading literature is a morally significant act. Living in a world marred by animosity and violence, a literary work provides a natural setting where one can uncover human interconnections and moral responsibilities. The experience of reading and the exposure to human otherness, according to Emmanuel Levinas, gives "access to the alterity of the Other" (121); it disturbs "the being at home with oneself" and provokes an ethical responsibility toward the other (39). Levinas' concepts of subjectivity, otherness, responsibility, and meaning motivate a critical reassessment of the ethical potentials inherent in literary texts. Confronted with narratives that portray characters with disabilities, therefore, ableist readers may experience cognitive dissonance when humanizing representations confront their preconceived stereotypes. This cognitive dissonance refers to the psychological tension that arises when alternative values and attitudes challenge the existing ones, serving as a catalyst for introspection (Caracciolo 22). Within this framework, the act of empathetic reading is an aesthetically immersive experience imbued with ethical implications. By immersing themselves in the emotions and thoughts of various characters, readers are able to broaden their understanding of other human beings and themselves.

Quayon's concept of "aesthetic nervousness" is also useful in the interpretation of Rushdie's *Shame* because the established modes of representation are disrupted in relation to disability. This disruption lies primarily in the conflicts between characters with and without disabilities, and it is further accentuated by the use of symbols, metaphors, and narrative techniques. In his analysis of autism in Coetzee's *Life and Times of Michael K*, Quayson writes:

> [...] the nature of the representation of cognitive disorders such as autism allows us to see the acute contradiction that is established within narrative between an implied interlocutor—shown here as a surrogate for the wider social domain—and the silent or inarticulate character who seems to opt for silence in negotiating the vicissitudes of social existence. The autistic character provides us with a template for seeing the relationship between speech and silence, and between the domain of cognitive disorder and that of social relations, where everyone is arguably spoken for within a social semiotic that cannot tolerate anomaly (much less silence). (147–148)

The quote reveals that the autistic character serves as a lens to examine the social rejection of "anomalies" and the notion that everyone is expected to conform to established norms.

Rushdie's *Shame* can eventually be read through the seventh type of Quayson's typology whereby disability carries an *"inarticulable and enigmatic tragic insight"* (49); it has an impenetrable meaning, and the character with a disability has a tragic flaw that is not easy to communicate. Sufiya is under the influence of a dialectical coupling of sorrowful comprehension and voice deprivation. The enigmatic and tragic aspects of her story are illustrated by the use of magic realism techniques, through which the author creates a kind of hallucination that is analogous to a nightmare. Magic realism operates beyond "the nature and limits of the knowable" to subvert the assumption "that reality is knowable, predictable, controllable" (Zamora and Faris 498). By combining realistic and fantastical elements to disrupt conventional understandings of reality, the magical realist representation of Sufiya urges readers to analyze the various levels of interpretation.

Conclusion

Rushdie's *Shame* has taken the metaphorical depiction of disability to an extraordinary level within the frame of magical realism, associating the disabled experience with feelings of shame and monstrousness. However, upon engaging in an empathetic interpretation, the human essence of the autistic character emerges, and the shame ultimately returns onto the ableist society. A fundamental question remains, however, unanswered. It is whether the author is perpetuating an ableist discourse or challenging readers to interrogate their own ableist prejudices to dismantle the social stigma surrounding disability. This question remains unanswered, reinforcing the idea that the novel has, in the words of Quayson, an *"inarticulable and enigmatic tragic insight"* (49).

3 "Aesthetic Nervousness" in John M. Coetzee's *Slow Man*

Introduction

This chapter examines John Maxwell Coetzee's *Slow Man* (2005) in respect to "the scar, the limp, the missing limb, or the obvious prosthesis" that "calls for a story" (Couser 457). The author demonstrates the distress of persons with disabilities in relation to issues of subjectivity, othering, aging, and caregiving. Using Quayson's concept of "aesthetic nervousness" and typology of disability representation, the chapter illustrates the relevance of type 1, *"Disability as null set and/or moral test"* (37) and type 2, *"Disability as the interface with otherness"* (39) in the understanding of the novel. As opposed to many global Anglophone writers who use amputation as a metaphor or "narrative prosthesis" (Mitchell and Snyder 49) for colonial violence and corporeal mutilation, Coetzee explores disability in its literal sense, illustrating the medical, social, and biopsychosocial models, with related institutional, interpersonal, and internalized forms of ableism.

"Disability as Null Set and Moral Test" vs. "Disability as the Interface with Otherness"

Quayson's *Aesthetic Nervousness: Disability and the Crisis of Representation* is a seminal book in the field of literary disability studies; this is even more so because his study includes illustrations from the broad field of global Anglophone literature. The idea he designates as "aesthetic nervousness" happens "when the dominant protocols of representation within the literary text are short-circuited in relation to disability" (15). It implies a deviation from the conventional norms of representation when it comes to portraying disability, and it constitutes a deliberate effort to disrupt traditional representations of disability to propose alternative narratives. "Aesthetic nervousness" resides primarily in the tensions between characters with and without disabilities, and it is magnified, at a secondary level, by the use of symbols, metaphors, and narrative devices. It can also find expression in the relationship between the reader and the literary text, as they discover the vicissitudes of characters with disabilities in relation to their social assumptions. Quayson contends that a typological classification of disability representations allows readers to probe into the literary work, noting that the nine types are not mutually exclusive. Coetzee's *Slow Man* lends itself to interpretations using the first type, "*Disability as null set and/or moral test*" (37), and the second one, "*Disability as the interface with otherness (race, class, sexuality, and social identity)*" (39), with multiple intersections between the two.

In Quayson's typology of disability representation, "*Disability as null set and/or moral test*" (37), the character with a disability functions not only as a catalyst for their self-discovery and self-empowerment, but also as a moral focal point for the other characters, acting as a means to evaluate or enhance their moral integrity. A character's disability "acts as some form of ethical background to the actions of other characters, or as a means of resisting or enhancing their moral standing" (36). The mathematical concept of "null set," in this sense, symbolizes the situation in which the character with a disability lacks an independent existence, and instead, functions as a conduit through which other characters can validate their abilities.

Paul Rayment, the protagonist of Coetzee's *Slow Man*, struggles with existential questions related to his disability, aging, and mortality, complicated by the absence of family caregivers. His leg was amputated after a bicycle accident, leading to his loss of agency, and he is no longer able to make decisions or take actions related to his own life. The situation leads him to question his own masculinity, saying, "A man not wholly a man, then: a half-man" (34); he even questions his humanity, saying, "If you have hitherto been a man, with a man's life, may you henceforth be a dog, with a dog's life. That is what the voice says, the voice out of the dark cloud" (26). He angrily complains about his reduced autonomy and increased solitude. Due to his disability, he is unable to find a compatible partner who meets the criteria he previously had; societal perceptions surrounding disability prevent him from getting the person his heart truly desires. He is rather compelled to pursue a relationship with someone who shares a similar condition of disability as dictated by ableist norms.

In Paul's interactions with otherness, the reader perceives ableism at different levels and in different forms. Ableism is defined as the prejudice, discrimination, and exclusion of persons with disabilities based on societal beliefs that consider them as inferior. At the institutional level, Paul is confronted with medical ableism, which is the principle that every form of disability requires "fixing," sometimes without taking into consideration the will of the person concerned (Nario-Redmond et al. 726). This medical model of disability perceives it as originating from an individual's physical impairment whose impact can be mitigated by "repairing" the body with pharmaceutical medications, surgical procedures, or other evidence-based therapies. At the interpersonal level, Paul faces ableism in his social relationships with people who fail to recognize his needs as a human being. For example, Elizabeth Costello[28] intrudes into the narrative to condemn the attraction of Paul toward a non-disabled woman as socially unacceptable. Instead, she suggests that he meet a blind woman who cannot see his amputated leg; she says, "Why not see what you can achieve together, you and Marianna, she blind, you halt?" (Coetzee 97). In this proposal, there is an assumption that two disabled bodies are suitable for each other.

At the institutional and social levels, therefore, as the previous examples show, ableism takes different forms. It can be hostile when the ableist displays aggressive behaviors towards an individual with a disability, benevolent when the ableist considers them as lacking strength and needing assistance, or ambivalent when the ableist combines both hostile and benevolent attitudes. The cumulative effect of institutional and social levels of ableism, with the different forms they take, leads Paul to an internalized level of ableism. In other words, "the processes of ableism, like those of racism, induce an internalisation or self-loathing which devalues disablement" (Campbell 20). In this regard, Paul reflects about Costello's proposal:

> Blindness is a handicap pure and simple. A man without sight is a lesser man, as a man without a leg is a lesser man, not a new man. This poor woman she has sent him is a lesser woman too, less than she must have been before. Two lesser beings, handicapped, diminished: how could she have imagined a spark of the divine would be struck between them, or any spark at all? (Coetzee 113)

This quote shows that Paul, despite his disability, displays ableist attitudes that derive from his internalized social responses to impairment. Otherness is becoming a part of his experience of disability.[29]

The second category in Quayson's typology of disability representation is *"Disability as the interface with otherness (race, class, sexuality, and social identity)"* (39), in which the person with a disability exhibits a noticeable corporeal disparity and moral deficiency that prompts other characters to recognize their own elevated standing. Quayson asserts, "Several disability scholars have already noted the

---

[28] Elizabeth Costello is a recurring character in Coetzee's works. She is the major character of the eponymous novel, *Elizabeth Costello*, but she intrudes into other novels like *The Lives of Animals* and *Slow Man* to provide ethical reflections.
[29] By definition, a person with a disability is one who has "long-term physical, mental, intellectual, or sensory impairments, which, in interaction with various barriers, may hinder their full and effective participation in society on an equal basis with others" (UNCRDP 4). In this definition, the issues surrounding disability extend beyond bodily functioning, highlighting the social preconceptions of normalcy and difference that have negative effects on persons with disabilities. This social model of disability addresses the barriers that impede their full inclusion, aiming to promote accessibility, inclusivity, and equality.

degree to which the disabled body sharply recalls to the nondisabled the provisional and temporary nature of able-bodiedness and indeed of the social frameworks that undergird the suppositions of bodily normality" (14). This quote indicates that the disabled body serves as a reminder to able-bodied individuals of the impermanent nature of their condition since nobody is exempt from the possibility of a disease or disability that may unexpectedly disrupt normal life.

Cure vs. Care

Immediately after his accident, Paul relies on external assistance to meet his most basic needs, and the hospital provides the healthcare he necessitates, but there are occasions when it transforms into a place of indifference and degradation. He complains, "It is only the pain, and the dragging, sleepless nights in this hospital, this zone of humiliation with no place to hide from the pitiless gaze of the young, that make him wish for death" (Coetzee 13). Paul's denunciation of the "pitiless gaze" recalls Michel Foucault's criticism of the "clinical gaze" in *The Birth of the Clinic: An Archaeology of Medical Perception*, in which he associates power, knowledge, and medical discourse. When a human being enters the hospital, their sickness is in search of a cure, Foucault argues, but it is "turned into a spectacle" under the domineering authority of the "clinical gaze" (85). He criticizes doctors for not being patient-oriented and denounces their dehumanizing mind-body dichotomy.

In a similar vein, Arthur Frank's *The Wounded Storyteller: Body, Illness, and Ethics* compares the practice of modern medicine to "colonialism." He contends, "Just as political and economic colonialism took over geographic areas, modernist medicine claimed the body of its patient as its territory" (10). For him, being a patient equates to "being colonized as medical territory and becoming a spectator to your own drama" (57). Frank's assertion, wherein the medical establishment assumes dominion over the body, relegates the patient to a passive observer of their own narrative. While there may be power dynamics within the healthcare system, this comparison seems to be an overstatement. The doctor commits to rescuing as much as possible from Paul's damaged leg (Coetzee 5), and the nurse confirms, "everything is taken care of" (4). They decide to amputate his leg and place a prosthesis; Paul is against the decision, saying, "I would prefer to take care of myself" (10), but his choice goes unheard. Until the end of the novel, his opinion does not change; "he dislikes prostheses, as he dislike all fakes" (255), but he is obliged to live in accordance with the doctor's will. The nurse advises him to "accept fate" (15) and curtails his hope of recovering his normalcy.

Coetzee's *Slow Man* establishes a contrast between cure and care, highlighting the difference between medical treatment aimed at healing the body and compassionate care aimed at nourishing the soul. The oxymoron of *indifferent care* intensifies Paul's sense of shame; he deplores the sight of *"indifferent* young people going through the motions of *caring* for him" (15), for his "curtailed" condition (14) of a "diminished man" (32). On his discharge, Mrs. Putts, the healthcare worker, proposes "a private nurse, someone with experience of frail care" (17). Her overbearing stance, rejected by Paul, represents "the welfare system" that cares "for people who cannot care for themselves" (22), but he is disconcerted by the nurses suggested to assist him in reprogramming his limb memories.

Due to the combination of his amputation, advanced age, and lack of familial ties, Paul has experienced a significant deprivation of his fundamental Basic Human Needs (BHN). Abraham Maslow's pyramid (see figure 13) categorizes these needs related to five distinct areas: physiology, security, society, esteem, and self-actualization. "Thwarting of unimportant desires," he believes, "produces no psychopathological results; thwarting of basically important needs does produce such results" (57). Paul possesses the necessary resources to meet most of his lower-level physiological needs, like water, food, and shelter, but he is unable to gratify his sexual drive toward the woman he loves. His security needs have for long been thwarted by the absence of family, but they have been complicated by his amputation and reduced professional activity. His disability also impedes the fulfillment of his social needs, mainly love and belonging, leading to a sense of isolation. In such conditions, meeting higher-level needs, such as esteem (self-esteem, respect), as well as self-actualization (the need to become what one is able to

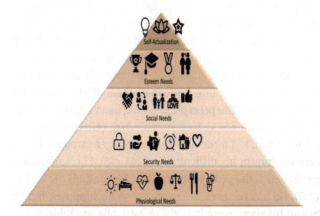

Figure 13: Abraham Maslow's Hierarchy of Basic Human Needs (author's design)

become), becomes almost impossible. With his Basic Human Needs being unmet, Paul's well-being and quality of life are gravely affected.

Paul, described as an "ageing cripple," needs "to be loved and to give love" (Coetzee 86); he needs a positive form of care, "not that dismaying and depressing prospect but this soft, consoling, and eminently feminine presence" (208). Elizabeth Costello makes a clearer distinction between love and care in these poignant words: "What we need is care: someone to hold our hand now and then when we get trembly, to make a cup of tea for us, help us down the stairs. Someone to close our eyes when the time comes" (154). In this sense, care seems to be a more important need than love. While love is an overarching emotion, care is a tangible manifestation of that emotion through actions that ensure the well-being of the loved person. Love can inspire care, and care can be a concrete way of expressing love.

Paul finds this need for care, rather than just cure, in Marijana, the Croatian private nurse. While Paul suffers from ableist attitudes of pity, condescension, and sometimes antagonism from healthcare providers, she is the only person who offers more empathetic healthcare that recognizes his humanity and dignity. Beyond massaging his back and tending to his stump (28), she takes on additional responsibilities such as shopping, cooking, and cleaning. Under her tender touch, Paul's "leg is day by day losing its angry colour and swollen look" (35). She also gives solace to the soul that resides in his ailing body; he understands that care is what he needs rather than cure. The narrator explains, "If there is any residue of belief in him, it has been shifted to Marijana Jokić, who […] promises no cure, just care" (63). He feels in her behavior a "loving care" that extends beyond the form of nursing driven by a sense of duty.

Marijuana's son, Drago, behaving like the son Paul does not have, helps him in his mother's absence. In a poignant scene, Paul urinates on the floor on his way to the bathroom; Drago assists the "helpless old man in urinous pyjamas trailing an obscene pink stump behind him from which sodden bandages are slipping" (214). In this particular example, Drago shows that the concept of care may not be driven by love, but it can adhere to a moral obligation. This is not, however, what Paul needs; he wants to adopt Drago. When he realizes that he must rely on caregivers for even the most insignificant tasks, including the management of his bladder, his deepest regret is the absence of a son. The perception of Marijana's appeal significantly emerges after Paul learns about her sixteen-year-old boy, reflecting his deep "regret that he does not have a son. […] a son and heir, a younger, stronger, better version of himself" to care for him in his difficult times (44–45). The amputation thus calls for a life review in which the protagonist realizes that "all his life he has been missing himself" (237). He has relatives in France, or so he supposes, but he lost touch with them; he and his sister were brought to Australia as children, but all of the family died (43). Without the comfort of relatives and friends, the grief of amputation cannot be stronger.

Coetzee's *Slow Man* explores, on a deeper ground, the relationship between disability and the ethics of reciprocal care. Paul needs non-physical, benevolent love and care that motivate him to provide for others. He insists, with reference to his inability to make love as he used to, "If I still practise love, I practise it in a different way" (144). After his accident, and during his life review process, he desires to make a positive impact by carrying out an action that could be, in his own words, a source of "blessing" in the lives of others. He wishes to provide this blessing to Marijana and her children by laying "a protective hand over them" (156). Having no possibility of offering other than material assistance, he sends her a letter in which he writes, "You have taken care of me; now I want to give something back, if you will let me. I offer to take care of you, or at least to relieve you of some of your burden. I offer to do so because in my heart, in my core, I care for you. You and yours" (165). Paul is fully prepared to offer whatever it takes to assume the role of a father to her children and to contribute financially to their education. In his new condition as a man with a disability, love is dressed with a new conception that signifies selflessness and benevolence.

Conclusion

The novel concludes on a relatively optimistic note as Paul overcomes his traumatic accident and finishes his rehabilitation. As readers observe the hardships he has faced, they undergo a "moral test" (Quayson 37). They may experience a sense of discomfort and question their own ableist attitudes, leading to empathy and tolerance. Coetzee's *Slow Man* obviously demonstrates the principle that "aesthetic nervousness" challenges readers to "lift [their] eyes from the reading of literature to attend more closely to the implications of the social universe around [them]" (Quayson 31). Central to the novel is Coetzee's criticism of the paternalistic model of doctor-patient relationships in which the doctor holds a position of authority over the "patient" whose experience of suffering[30] puts them in a subaltern position. Implied in this is a call for a therapeutic alliance centered on the care seeker, with respect for their humanity and acceptance of their active participation in decision-making. The poignant message is ultimately that persons with disabil-

---

[30] Etymologically, "patient" is derived from the Latin word "patior," meaning "to suffer." See Julia Neuberger's "Do we Need a New Word for Patients? Lets do Away with 'Patients.'" *BMJ (Clinical research ed.)*, vol. 318, no. 7200, 1999, pp. 1756–1757. www.ncbi.nlm.nih.gov/pmc/articles/PMC1116090/pdf/1756.pdf. Accessed 10 Apr. 2022.

ities are more than impaired limbs and persistent symptoms; they are whole human beings with the same longings and apprehensions as other human beings.

Part V: **Holistic Healing in the Global Anglophone Novel**

1 Autopathography and the Healing Garden in Bessie Head's *A Question of Power*

Introduction

Bessie Head's *A Question of Power* (1973) is an autopathography, or illness narrative, that foregrounds the author's own tussle with madness. It seems to be structurally bipolar, as it starts with a dystopian picture of the apartheid in South Africa and its toll on Elizabeth's sanity. The novel eventually provides an alternative nature-based treatment in which the garden serves as a sanctuary, a metaphor for the protagonist's own journey of healing and transformation. Just as she carefully tends to her plants and nurtures them to health, she learns to nurture herself and cultivate her own emotional resilience.

Autopathographic Exploration of Madness

The term "pathography" is derived from the Greek words "pathos," meaning suffering, and "graphia," meaning writing. "Autopathography" is a form of autobiographical writing where the author recounts their personal journey with the disease, including diagnosis, treatment, and quality of life. It can cover a wide range of conditions, including physical diseases such as cancer or HIV/AIDS, as well as mental health issues like depression or schizophrenia. In her work "Pathography: Patient Narratives of Illness," Anne H. Hawkins argues that pathographies give voice to the worries and aspirations related to disease, and serve as reference books about lived experiences. Hawkins provides the following typology: The first one is "didactic pathography" that teaches about a given disease, like breast cancer or HIV/AIDS, by blending "practical information" with personal narrative. The second type is "angry pathography" that is driven by personal disappointments about deficiencies in the healthcare system like the healthcare professionals' lack of empathy. The third type is "alternative pathography" that shares the disappointment evoked in the previous type and proposes some alternative treatments. The fourth type is "ecopathography" that connects the individual experience of disease to broader environmental issues. For patients, pathographies facilitate recovery through writing; for caregivers and the general readership, they enhance empathy and provide clues for dealing with one's own disease or the disease of a loved one. For healthcare professionals, in addition to nurturing empathy, they provide valuable knowledge about patients' experiences through detailed case studies, with examples of how the delivery of bad news and expressions of empathy affect the lives of patients and their families (127–129).

What is striking is that Head's *A Question of Power* seems to cover the four types of pathographies. It is didactic because it teaches readers about madness, blending her personal accounts of the disease with practical information on how to cope with it. It also belongs to the angry type because the author expresses her disappointment about the disparities and dehumanizing experiences in the apartheid system. It also falls under the third category because it offers alternative treatments like gardening therapy. Finally, it is an ecopathography because it shows the importance of the environment in the treatment of mental disorders.

Elizabeth, the protagonist of *A Question of Power*, was born from an affair between a white woman and an unknown black man, a legally forbidden union back in the 1930s. During her pregnancy, the mother was placed in the mental hospital where the author was born. The mother allegedly committed suicide thereafter, and the author was adopted by a black woman. When she grew up, she was given a letter in which her mother asked, "Please set aside some money for my child's education" (16), raising questions about the possibility of an insane person to write a letter and a will like this one, and implying that other people labeled her as insane, and probably murdered her. There is no explicit evidence suggesting that the mother was genuinely mentally ill, and the individuals who claimed her madness are those belonging to the apartheid institution who intended to influence Elizabeth into presuming her inherent insanity. The mother's insanity, so to speak, more likely lies in her breach of South Africa's Immorality Amendment Act of 1957 that prohibited interracial relationships.

Elizabeth is therefore a "tragic mulatta," a mixed-race woman who experiences a tragic life because of her apartheid society. The apartheid (1948–1994) was a government-sanctioned system of racial segregation that maintained white minority rule, enforcing strict socioeconomic and political separation between different racial groups. The system institutionalized racial inequality and denied basic human rights to the majority of the population, perpetuating systemic oppression, racial tensions, and social unrest. It came to an end with the dismantling of discriminatory laws and the election of Nelson Mandela as South Africa's first black President in 1994.

Elizabeth's madness is both the result of a racist colonial society and a strategy of survival and resistance. Her major traumatic event happens when, in her childhood, the school principal refers to some records that label her as potentially insane due to her mother's affair with an African stable boy. The experience leads her to internalize the belief in her inherent inclination towards madness. The school principal's voice keeps haunting her days and nights through unconscious flashbacks, episodes of panic or rage, and awful nightmares: "your mother was a white woman. They had to lock her up, as she was having a child by the stable boy, who was a native" (16). In these nightmares, Elizabeth perceives herself as lacking a vagina, beheaded, or mutilated; she also encounters deceased individuals and large, sexually deviant men.

The structure of the novel exhibits a bipolar nature. The sections that focus on Elizabeth's inner world are characterized by darkness, devastation, and death imagery whereas the sections that focus on her external reality portray her engaged in the healing act of gardening. Her involvement in gardening exposes her to the remarkable peculiarities of human nature and the vibrant vitality of lush green vegetation (Pearse 88). The author's proficiency in expressing the symbolic language of madness in *A Question of Power* stems from the fusion of her own mental disease and her fascination with psychoanalysis. Drawing upon the psychoanalysts' division of the human mind into the conscious, subconscious, and unconscious, she vividly captures her protagonist's journey, showing the significance of childhood experiences in the mental constitution of the individual. Medusa, Sello and Dan, dwell in her dreams and nightmares to communicate not only prophecies about her madness, death, and her son's murder, but also philosophies about love, humanity, and healing. They are not human characters but representations in Elizabeth's mind. These eerie figures, perceptible solely to her, personify her innermost self, namely her subconscious and unconscious realms. Sello personifies her subconscious, which is deeply flawed but endowed with a belief in goodness. Dan and Medusa, however, personify the malevolent forces and power dynamics in South African society; they urge her to commit suicide, but she refuses to comply with their commands.

Cultivating Sanity in the Edenic Garden

In "Biophilia: Does Visual Contact with Nature Impact on Health and Well-Being?" Bjorn Grinde and Grete G. Patil observe that, owing to the natural conception of the human mind, the lack of contact with nature creates "a discord." They therefore argue that a regained contact with nature enhances mental health; using the concept of "biophilia," innate love for the natural world, they explain, "According to the concept of discords, a positive effect suggests that those who presently obtain a suboptimal dose of exposure to plants have a concomitantly reduced life quality. Current statistics of mental health do not contradict this model" (2334). Long before the concept of ecopsychology and biophilia emerged, various forms of horticulture therapy have been used for centuries, as human beings have recognized the therapeutic benefits of engaging with farming and gardening, providing solace through the connection with the natural world.

In his seminal article titled "Effects of Gardens on Health Outcomes: Theory and Research," Roger Ulrich proposes his theory of "supportive garden design" in which he claims improved health outcomes if patients are exposed to healing gardens. He identifies four potential benefits: Firstly, spending time in natural surroundings is often associated with physical activity, which is clearly beneficial for one's health. Secondly, engaging in nature-related activities frequently involves socializing, such as walking or gathering with friends in a park, which has positive effects on well-being. Thirdly, nature provides an opportunity to temporarily break away from everyday routines and responsibilities, offering a refreshing escape (36). Ulrich also reports that having a window with a view of trees reduces the need for pain medication and hospital stays ("View through a Window" 224).

Tom Holzinger, a Bessie Head Heritage Trust member, describes Head's real-life garden as productive and fruitful. She cultivated a diverse array of plants, including gooseberry bushes for making and selling jam; she collected seeds and explored different plant species (Wolff). Apart from maintaining her home garden, Head also played a role in establishing a communal garden in Serowe[1] where she collaborated with other volunteers on a shared piece of land. In *A Question of Power*, when she is no longer capable of dealing with the maddening circumstances in South Africa, Elizabeth seeks asylum in Botswana, looking for quietude. There, she meets Eugene, the co-op chief and mentor, an Afrikaner who also left South Africa to devote himself to assisting displaced individuals and building an alternative society. Understanding the reason why "South Africans usually suffered from some form of mental aberration" (58), he tells Elizabeth that "too much isolation isn't a good thing" (56), and he invites her to join his cooperative gardening project where she finally feels a sense of belonging. He becomes a role model of resilience who teaches her that one can only strive to experience love by embracing humility and making sacrifices, and that love is an act of giving, not of taking or anticipating reciprocation.

The healing garden materializes Head's philosophy of diversity and inclusivity, as the gardeners are from South African, American, English, and Danish origins. Elizabeth engages in gardening and marketing fresh produce within her village, forming connections with admirable individuals from the community. Through their communal gardening, Elizabeth develops a closer bond with human beings. She finds herself surrounded by a supportive group of individuals who assist her in her transformation and broaden her understanding of the world. Working, sharing, and laughing with others is an entirely novel experience for her. Tom, the white American, plays a particular role in Elizabeth's metamorphosis through

---

1 See Head's novel *Serowe: Village of the Rain Wind.* Heinemann, 1981.

his compassionate listening skills; he changes the initial animosity toward white people she had earlier formed in the apartheid society. She frequently confides in him, discussing her mental health afflictions, philosophical musings, and perspectives on life. She asks him, "Tom, you like to take care of people. Will you take care of me the way you care for others?" He answers her with "intensity: 'Willingly'" (136). This meeting with humans who care restores Elizabeth's broken connections, and she feels empowered in a way she has never experienced before.

Elizabeth successfully cultivates an array of vegetables in her garden, including massive cabbage, Cape gooseberries, and spinach. Both the local villagers in Motabeng and foreigners from England appreciate her gardening achievements, showing she has regained the ability to be productive. Much to her happiness, "the village women always passed by Elizabeth's house to collect firewood in the bush. If they saw her in the yard, they stopped, laughed and said: 'Cape Gooseberry' [...] they did it so often that eventually Elizabeth became known as 'Cape Gooseberry'" (153). In "Cape Gooseberries and Giant Cauliflowers: Transplantation, Hybridity, and Growth in Bessie Head's *A Question of Power*," Anissa Talahite considers the garden as Head's endeavor to "redefine the relationship between the social world and the individual self" (141). She analyzes how Elizabeth cultivates Cape gooseberry, a fruit of South African origins whose seeds she has planted in her garden, placing emphasis not on the result but on the collective process of planting seeds. In this perspective, the novel employs gardening as a metaphor for cross-cultural connections in post-apartheid South Africa.

Consequently, and in contrast to her own mother, Elizabeth thrives and nurtures her son. While her mother has, allegedly, succumbed to insanity and committed suicide, Elizabeth grapples with suicidal thoughts but refuses to succumb to them. In this manner, "by turning inwards," Elizabeth realizes that "the centre of herself was still sane and secure, and that the evils which had begun to dominate her mind had a soaring parallel of goodness. It seemed to be all that mattered, a reassurance of goodness that was a still, steady, deathless flame" (Head 55). This quote reflects Elizabeth's introspective journey and realization that, despite her internal struggles, there exists a core within her that remains remarkably sane and inherently good. In her discussion with a friend called Birgette, Elizabeth relates a vision in which she is overwhelmed with an extraordinary potential of love, saying, "I have a peculiar sensation of sleeping with a whole lot of people in my arms, like a great and eternal mother. I thought: Love is so powerful, it's like unseen flowers under your feet as you walk" (86). Eventually, she subverts the "power people" who feed on "other people's souls like vultures" (19). Despite the dark sides of her human existence, the tormented mind discovers a glimmer of optimism; the hell of loneliness and segregation in South Africa eventually contrasts with the Eden of community and serenity in Botswana.

Conclusion

Bessie Head's *A Question of Power* is deeply rooted in the historical context of South Africa and Botswana, as well as the broader history of colonialism in Africa and its relation to mental health. Gardening plays a significant role in the main character's journey of self-discovery and healing; it stands as a powerful symbol of the transformative power of nature, as well as the importance of finding a sense of connection to the natural world. Despite her insanity, Elizabeth emerges from her story as a more humane and knowledgeable person; the initiation of Sello and Dan teaches her the hard way about suffering, power, and humanity.

2 Curative Eco-narrative in Leslie Marmon Silko's *Ceremony*

Introduction

Leslie Marmon Silko's *Ceremony* (1977) is a Native American narrative of communal eco-recovery. Curative eco-narrative plays a major role in the healing of the Native American protagonist, Tayo, a World War II veteran who is suffering from Post-Traumatic Stress Disorder and cultural displacement. His grandmother and other members of his community use storytelling to help him understand his place in the world, in relation to his culture and his land. In 1973, in the context of anti-Vietnam War sentiment, Silko traveled with her husband to Alaska, a completely different place from her native desert in New Mexico; the displacement acted as a turning point in her life and influenced her literary career. In an interview with Dexter Fisher, she reveals that writing *Ceremony* "was a cure for what appears to be not just Tayo's but her own tussle with madness," and "As Tayo got better, [she] got better" (20). The novel is a testimonial logotherapeutic (Frankl 140) and scriptotherapeutic (Henke xi) narrative, inspired by the storytelling tradition that celebrates the healing power of the wise word and the natural world.

The Gynocratic Custody of Eco-healing Traditions

Native American communities emphasize the healing power of Mother/Nature. In *The Sacred Hoop: Recovering the Feminine in American Indian Traditions*, Paula Gunn Allen describes them as gynocratic, i.e., "woman-centered tribal societies in which matrilocality, matrifocality, matrilinearity, maternal control of household goods and resources [...] were and are present and active features of traditional tribal life" (3–4). With European settlements, however, the roles of women were reduced to childbearing, rearing, and domestic chores because the invaders "could not tolerate peoples who allowed women to occupy prominent positions and decision-making capacity at every level of society" (3). The redistribution of gender roles shook the foundation of communal structure, but in contemporary Native American literature, women are revived as sustainers of communal solidarity and agents of change. They are also the preservers of healing traditions, secret keepers of herbal medicines, and ritual ceremonies. Women have an essential position in the organization of the family and the tribe, a position maintained principally through their power to tell stories. A powerful female archetype constitutes "the backbone" of oral traditions, like Spider Woman for the Navajo, Sky Woman for the Iroquois, and Corn Daughter for the Hopi. In the Laguna Pueblo mythology, Spider Woman, Yellow Woman, or Thought Woman, is the creatrix, the weaver of the "Web of life." Silko explains that "human identity, imagination, and storytelling were inextricably linked to the land, to Mother Earth, just as strands of the spider's web radiate from the center of the web" (*Yellow* 21). By weaving the web, the spider symbolizes creative power and convergence towards the center; by analogy, the ecosystem is like a spider web: if one strand is broken, the whole is affected.

Tightly related to the importance of women in ecofeminist terms is the importance of the land. Silko wrote her novel in a period when environmental justice activists started a global campaign against the environmental destruction of the habitats in which Indigenous peoples live. The earliest nuclear tests occurred on Native American lands where serious diseases are presently diagnosed; native "lands are subject to some of the most invasive industrial interventions imaginable. According to the Worldwatch Institute, 317 reservations in the United States are threatened by environmental hazards, ranging from toxic wastes to clearcuts" (LaDuke 2). Los Alamos Laboratory in New Mexico, for instance, is situated in a Pueblo area, and it is the place where weapons of mass destruction have been manufactured and tested, like the Hiroshima and Nagasaki atomic bombs (Kutler 222). An important radioactive leak also occurred on the Navajo reservation in 1978. Ecologists and historians use the expression "radioactive colonialism" to characterize the placement of Native Americans in radioactive "sacrifice zones" where uranium is mined, waste is dumped, and bombs are tested (Grinde and Johansen 3). Ashlee Cunsolo and Neville R. Ellis use the concept of "ecological grief" to explain the human feeling "in relation to experienced or anticipated ecological losses, including the loss of species, ecosystems, and meaningful landscapes due to acute or chronic environmental change" (275). This concept encompasses the sense of sorrow that individuals and communities feel in response to environmental degradation, as well as the significant impact it has on human well-being. It reflects the deep connection between human beings and their natural environment and calls for consequential awareness and action in the face of environmental challenges.

To treat this "ecological grief," as well as their traumatic grief, Native Americans believe in the healing power of the word. For them, bodily illness reflects spiritual unbalance and loss of harmony with the universe. Those who suffer from what shamans call "soul loss" seek "soul restoration" and communal reconnection by means of ceremonies that bind the sick to the wellspring of tribal energy. Ceremonies, in this sense, "hold the society together, create harmony, restore balance, ensure prosperity and unity, and establish right relations within the social and natural world" (Allen, "The Sacred Hoop" 259). This holistic approach to healing combines the treatment of the body, the mind, and the soul; the shaman intervenes as a link with the spirit world of animals, plants, and inanimate objects in order to mend the broken connections. He employs different methods to enter an altered state of consciousness, like dancing to the rhythm of drums and ingesting hallucinogenic substances, emphasizing the healing potentials of symbolic and metaphoric representations in ritual ceremonies.

The Etiology of Tayo's Illness

In Siko's *Ceremony*, Tayo's illness starts with his participation in World War II. Like many Native Americans, he enlists in the army with the hope of escaping from the poverty of the reservation since the government promises them the opportunity to be integrated into mainstream American society. Hope soon turns into disenchantment, and Tayo returns from the war with a severe "battle fatigue" (8). He suffers from Post-Traumatic Stress Disorder (PTSD), particularly survivor guilt, the mental disorder of an individual who feels guilty for surviving a traumatic event while relatives or friends died. He survived the Bataan Death March (April 9, 1942) in the Philippines whereas his cousin Rocky perished. The sense of guilt experienced by Tayo illustrates the "response, sometimes delayed, to an overwhelming event or events, which takes the form of repeated, intrusive hallucinations, dreams, thoughts, or behaviors stemming from the event" (Caruth 4). Childhood recollections of his Uncle Josiah's pleasant storytelling and his cousin Rocky's playful companionship disintegrate into the appalling images of their deaths during the war.

One of the veterans, called Emo, is the embodiment of what Silko calls "witchery" in this novel to describe Euro-American imperialism on a global scale. Bragging about the number of Japanese people he murdered, Emo says, "we butchered every Jap we found. No Jap bastard was fit to take prisoner" and "we blew them all to hell. We should've dropped bombs on all the rest and blown them off the face of the earth." He then rattles a bag of teeth that he "knocked out of the corpse of a Japanese soldier" (Silko, *Ceremony* 60–61). Emo believes that being pitilessly violent with the enemy of the USA is the only way to get a good position in society, even if the cost is his loss of human feelings. Tayo vomits whenever he hears the rattle of teeth in Emo's bag; this is the major symptom of his illness, as if his belly is trying to purge itself of some poison, probably the poison of "white lies" that set him in a position of worthlessness in the web of life. In "Knotted Bellies and Fragile Webs: Untangling and Re-Spinning in Tayo's Healing Journey," Jude Todd counts the appearance of the word "belly" no less than "once on 71 of the 262 pages" of the novel, and the word bears the "great swollen grief that was pushing into his throat" (9). In his attempt to keep his stomach "unknotted," Tayo finds refuge in alcohol with other veterans who try "to sink the loss in booze" (169). Thinking that "Liquor was medicine [...] for tight bellies and choked-up throats" (40), Tayo gets sicker. To be healed, he needs to purge his belly of the lies he has been ingesting since his childhood, that his mother was blameworthy because she had conceived him with a white man, that his ancestral traditions were full of irrationality, and that he was fighting for a just cause in WWII.

By night, Tayo usually wakes up in a sweat, feeling "inside his skull the tension of little threads being pulled and how it was with tangled things, things tied together, and as he tried to pull them apart and rewind them into their places, they snagged and tangled even more." He sweats at the idea that something "wasn't unraveled or tied in knots to the past–something that existed by itself, standing alone like a deer" (Silko, *Ceremony* 6–7). This passage reflects the loneliness that takes a toll on Tayo's mind, and his vomiting is a psychosomatic symptom of this ailing. The nexus between the body and the mind is illustrated in the old man's observation:

> I will tell you something about stories [...] They aren't just entertainment. [...] They are [...] all we have to fight off / illness and death. [...] He rubbed his belly. / I keep them here [...] Here, put your hand on it / See, it is moving. / There is life here for the people. / And in the belly of this story / the rituals and the ceremony / are still growing. (2)

The belly is the place where Spider Woman, too, keeps her stories. This symbolism suggests that the stories are not just external but deeply internalized entities within each individual.

After a fight with Emo in a surge of anger, Tayo is taken to a psychiatric ward where he describes his state to the psychiatrist as follows, "He cries all the time. Sometimes he vomits [...] He cries because they are dead and everything is dying [...] He is invisible. His words [...] have no sound" (15–16). In this example, Tayo uses the pronouns "he" and "his" instead of "I" and "my," showing that his identity crisis is associated with inarticulateness; he is unable to identify with his own self, his perception of which is one of "white smoke" with "no consciousness of itself" (14). He associates the whiteness of walls, sheets, and uniforms with the whiteness of the dominant society and its "medicine [that] drained memory out of his thin arms and replaced it with a twilight cloud behind his eyes" (15). This example brings to mind the importance of holistic healing environments in healthcare settings. After weeks of worrisome non-recovery and desperate loneliness, Tayo asks for his grandmother. On the edge of his hospital bed, she lilts, "Those white doctors haven't helped you at all"; she puts his head on her lap and repeatedly says in tears, "A'moo'oh[31], a'moo'ohh" (33). This Laguna word of endearment welcomes Tayo back into the warm embrace of his community.

Despite the recognition that Tayo's case is a "mystery" to his scientific knowledge, the psychiatrist forbids him to take any "Indian medicine" (31) and "that he had to think only of himself and not about the others, that he would never get well as long as he used words like 'we' and 'us' " (125). The psychiatrist's attempts to cure Tayo with biomedical treatments are to no avail; yet, he prevents him from seeking ethnomedical alternatives. In fact, the "western trauma model does not acknowledge spirituality as a reference point; indeed, it denies the possibility of regeneration through ritual and belief systems" (Visser 279). While earlier treatment of trauma was usually based on empirical and evidence-based medicine, there has been an increasing interest among postcolonial trauma theorists and therapists in the potential benefits of spirituality in trauma recovery. In this regard, Fanon's work was revolutionary in the 1950s. Starting from the premise that "the biological, the psychological, the sociological were only separated by an aberration of the mind" (Fanon and Azoulay 363), he practiced sociotherapy (social therapy) that he had learned from François Tosquelle at Saint-Alban asylum in France. The method creates a miniature society inside the mental asylum, and it involves, in Fanon and Azoulay's conception, the treatment of the medical establishment before the treatment of the care seeker. It was a groundbreaking psychiatric practice in a colonial hospital in the Algerian city of Blida, as Fanon encouraged some activities like gardening, sports, and music. He additionally recognized the importance of spirituality in healthcare and allowed the regular visits of Muslim priests and storytellers. As it will be explained in Silko's *Ceremony*, trauma is treated through a sociotherapeutic approach despite the white psychiatrist's insistence to avoid "Indian medicine."

Tayo's Ceremonial Rite of Eco-recovery

For Native Americans, physical illness is a symptom of spiritual disharmony and disconnection from the web of life; those afflicted by what shamans call "soul loss" actively seek "soul restoration" through communal and environmental reconnection. Through transformative ceremonies, the sick are bound to the wellspring of tribal energy, a process that binds communities, restores equilibrium, fosters unity, and nurtures harmonious relationships with all creations (Allen, "The Sa-

---

[31] "A'moo'oh" is an expression of endearment in the Keresan language of the Laguna Pueblo people.

cred Hoop" 259). This holistic approach to healing integrates the well-being of the body, mind, and soul, with the help of shamans who serve as intermediaries with the spirit world of animals, plants, and inanimate objects to mend the severed bonds. The phrase *"mitakuye oyasin"* (all my relations) is the guiding principle of these ritual ceremonies, in which the shaman relies on the healing power of symbolic representations (Modaff 341). For Native Americans, therefore, the land is not only a means of sustenance, but also the witness of their history and the definer of their identity, as it embraces the bones of their ancestors.

Silko's *Ceremony* belongs to a type of writing recently categorized as "ecosickness fiction" which imaginatively views the link between the sick body and environmental consciousness. In *Ecosickness in Contemporary U.S. Fiction: Environment and Affect*, Heather Houser contends that "it is impossible to approach somatic and ecological inquiry as isolated phenomena" (224). Nature has the power to evoke a range of emotional responses that influence human affect in various ways. On the one hand, exposure to natural settings often induces positive feelings such as tranquility, awe, and well-being; on the other hand, environmental degradation may lead to negative affective states, including stress and anxiety. Tayo's family realizes that, to cure his ecosickness, he needs an Indigenous healing solution that the white psychiatrist is unable to provide; his grandmother says, "The only cure / I know / is a good ceremony" (Silko, *Ceremony* 3). For the Native American shaman, what Tayo needs is a ceremony that takes him on a journey back to his origins and forward into the path of healing. His disease is "part of something larger, and his cure would be found only in something great and inclusive of everything" (126). Paula Gunn Allen explains that "healing chants and ceremonies emphasize restoration of wholeness, for disease is a condition of division and separation from the harmony of the whole" (*The Sacred Hoop* 117). In the same vein, Linda Hogan defines ceremony as "the mending of a broken connection" between human beings and the rest of Creation. The participant pronounces the phrase "All my relations" which "create a relationship with other people, with animals, with the land" (40). In this way, Tayo needs to recover his internal peace by piecing together his shattered self, establishing harmonious bonds with the human and more-than-human communities.

Although women and their stories constitute the "backbone" of Native society, the two male shamans, Ku'oosh and Betonie, play a major role in Tayo's healing; they constitute a basic starting point for his reconnection to the tribal land. He feels better whenever Ku'oosh gives him herbal medicines, including tea and blue cornmeal, to soothe his stomach. He also feels good whenever he teaches him the older language of his people, telling him that "this world is fragile" (Silko, *Ceremony* 35) like a spider web shot by the sun, and that one person can "tear away the delicate strands of the web, spilling the rays of the sun into the sand" and harming the whole world (38). Betonie, in turn, uses Indigenous paraphernalia like dried tobacco, healing herbs, and gourd rattles; he initiates the healing ceremony by informing Tayo about the names of sacred places in the Native culture. He advises him to go to the place "where whirling darkness started its journey" (142), meaning that the treatment of trauma depends on the confrontation with the evil that caused it. Betonie sets up a curative sand painting, a sweat lodge ceremony (see figure 14), and a vision quest, adopting a holistic approach to well-being and emphasizing self-discovery through interconnectedness with the universe.

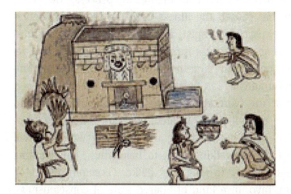

Figure 14: The Sweat Lodge Ceremony: Pre-Columbian Mesoamerican Temazcal (Public domain image from *Codex Magliabechiano*, reproduced from Fields 10)

Betonie outlines a curative sandpainting that represents Tayo's ritual ceremony, informing him that he should recover his uncle's stolen cattle, go to the mountain, and meet a woman. This sandpainting is a mandala that has different names in different Native American tribes, like the "medicine wheel" or the "sacred hoop"; it represents the universe, unity, wholeness, eternity, birth, death, and rebirth. In their *Handbook of Native American Mythology*, Dawn Bastian and Judy Mitchell maintain, "The power of Navajo sandpainting is in the merging of time and space into a place where the present and the mythic past coexist." Through associated ceremonial rituals, the "individual can be transported to a place where the present and the mythic world are one, a place where supernatural assistance and healing can be found" (36). The mandala, as a reproduction of the basic elements of creation and existence, provides a refuge for Indigenous people and a means of achieving wholeness. The quaternary shape stands for the "axis mundi" (axis of the world) that provides healing in contrast to the "axis of evil" that caused the illness. In *Myth and Reality*, Mircea Eliade explains, "The mandala is primarily an imago mundi [image of the world]; it represents the cosmos in miniature and, at the same time, the pantheon. Its construction is equivalent to a magical re-creation of the world." He considers that ritual practices that involve mandalas have "a therapeutic purpose. Made symbolically contemporary with the Creation of the World, the patient is immersed in the primordial fullness of life; he is penetrated by the gigantic forces that, in illo tempore, made the Creation possible" (25). For Eliade, ceremonial rituals through mandalas have a healing and transformative power by allowing the individual to be immersed in a sacred and symbolic reenactment of the primordial moment of creation.

Through the sandpainting, Betonie goes back with Tayo, like a psychotherapist, "to the origin of his being, to renew his energy for the healing process." He listens to him talking about the evil that caused the illness until the "guilty burden is somehow relieved." Unlike the psychotherapist, however, Betonie uses rituals and symbols "to mediate the renewal process through symbols of death and rebirth" (Sandner 245), ultimately positioning him in a novel and reconstructed universe where humans and non-humans live in harmony. A major aspect of this ceremony is the healing power of the word through the recitation of chants and prayers. Tayo's trauma needs to be holistically treated: physically, mentally, emotionally, and spiritually; Betonie asks him to recite the following words: "I will bring you through my hoop [...] I'm walking back to belonging / I'm walking home to happiness / I'm walking back to long life" (Silko, *Ceremony* 143–144). The chants and prayers orient Tayo, in a kind of altered state of consciousness, through mythical time to piece together his fragmented memories.

By virtue of his ritual ceremony, Tayo should first cut the fence of a private property to get his uncle's cattle back, but he feels like a thief before realizing that he is just recovering what was earlier stolen from his uncle. He remembers the widely believed "lie" that "only brown-skinned people were thieves; white people didn't steal, because they always had the money to buy whatever they wanted" (191). He understands how deeply such lies have been ingrained in people's minds and how much they are part of the "witchery" he is on his way to fight. While cutting the fence, he thinks about the other Native properties that whites have stolen, as they have taken Native lands for the sake of Manifest Destiny and Native children for the sake of assimilationist education. Tayo finally recovers the spotted cattle, with brown-and-white patterns on their hide. They are like him, a crossbreed between a brown and a white race, with a hybrid vigor that makes them adaptive survivors.

Whole Again with the Human and the More-than-human Worlds

Tayo's trauma is initially depicted in terms of a tangled spider web; he "could feel it inside his skull–the tension of little threads being pulled [...] things tied together, and as he tried to pull them apart and rewind them into their places, they snagged and tangled even more" (7). The Pueblos use a very suggestive image to illustrate this view of interconnectedness as a spider web whose weaving is so delicate that when a thread is broken, the entire fabric is damaged. Symbolically, they often pull threads from the fabric of their clothes when they are about to tell a story, and by analogy, in their view, when the bonds between the individual, the community, and nature are broken, the entire cosmic balance is disturbed.

Tayo's healing depends on Spider Woman the creatrix who disentangles his life by weaving stories of healing around him. She appears to him in the form of different female characters who guide him towards healing, not only his grandmother, but also his lover Ts'eh Montaño, the embodiment of Spider Woman or Yellow Woman of Laguna mythology. When he arrives at the mountain, viewed as "axis mundi," readers realize that they have entered mythical time. Ts'eh is wearing a yellow skirt, standing under an apricot tree, surrounded by yellow corn, flowers, and pollen. As an herbalist healer who lives close to the sacred land, her role is to reconnect the male protagonist to his Laguna land and culture; she is the "matrix" of the gynocratic system that would ultimately heal him.

Ts'eh feeds Tayo with dried corn like a loving mother, which symbolizes not only sustenance, but also the origin of the tribe. The idyllic setting of the mountain illustrates Ts'eh's ritual initiation of Tayo, reconnecting him to his ancestral landscape and showing him Indigenous curative roots and plants. Ts'eh, who stands for the land from an ecofeminist lens, fills Tayo's "hollow spaces with new dreams" (219), and their sexual encounters are depicted in ritual terms, like ceremonies of the Earth that resituate the protagonist at the center of his Laguna culture. After this ceremonial ritual, Tayo meets his former fellow veterans drinking with a Native woman; he does not join the group because he has understood the mechanisms of white manipulation (158). He tries to convince them that they have internalized their own oppression, but a fight suddenly starts and Tayo wants to kill Emo. He soon realizes that this action would once again destroy him spiritually; the narrator explains, "the witchery had almost ended the story according to its plan" because Tayo "had almost jammed the screwdriver into Emo's skull the way the witchery had wanted" (253). Silko's ending highlights the destruction that Tayo has finally overcome, and announces, "the witchery is dead *for now*" (261, emphasis added). Even though this is a happy denouement, "for now" implies circumspection to prevent the recrudescence of the "witchery."

A feeling of serenity overwhelms Tayo for not surrendering to the drive of destruction thanks to Ts'eh's initiation; he slumbers and dreams of being "wrapped in a blanket" in a wagon with his relatives; "they were taking him home" (254). This dream signals the end of the rite of passage and the hero's reintegration into his community. The novel ends while Tayo is crossing "the river at sunrise" (255), connoting a movement forward in the life cycle, purification, and resurrection. Motion at the end of the ceremony is a symbol of healing; as opposed to Tayo's earlier stasis in the psychiatric ward, he ultimately goes home, passing through hoops, doorways, and turning around "sunwise." Since the sun is a symbol of life, light, and energy, a sunwise movement aligns with the natural order, promoting harmony and energy.

Conclusion

Writing like a spider who spins a web, Silko insists on the redemptive power of the wise word and the natural world, as she makes women the locus of power and regeneration. Women are not only fundamental for the protagonist's healing, but also for the continuing lifecycle that allows the survival of the community and the conservation of Nature. The protagonist's grandmother is the first provider of support through her stories that act as healing narratives for his psychic wounds. Ts'eh is his second helper who overwhelms him with love and guidance to resist the destructive influence of evil. With the help of the powerful female archetype and the male shamans that reconcile him with all his relations, "*mitakuye oyasin*," Tayo goes through a journey from illness, loneliness, and despair towards health, reconnection, and hope.

3 Eco-artistic Recovery in Delia Jarrett-Macauley's *Moses, Citizen and Me*

Introduction

The focus of this chapter is on the eco-artistic recovery of traumatized child soldiers in Delia Jarrett-Macauley's *Moses, Citizen and Me* (2005). The novel uses the arts – storytelling, drama, music, song, and dance – in the natural environment of the forest as an approach to the treatment of war trauma. The recovery process relies on a variety of methods led by Julia and Bemba G. who try to reconcile child soldiers with themselves and their communities. The children need to regain control over their lives, and to begin the healing process, they need to voice their traumatic stories in safe ways. Julia and Bemba G. teach them the importance of self-reflection, creativity, communication, and collaboration in the process of recovery; they equally coach them to overcome their harrowing past, inviting them to become active agents in their healing journey and to move forward in life peacefully.

Child Soldiers' War Trauma

The trauma of child soldiers is an important theme in global Anglophone fiction, especially African fiction, with major works like Ken Saro-Wiwa's *Sozaboy* (1994), Ahmadou Kourouma's *Allah Is not Obliged* (2000), Uzodinma Iweala's *Beasts of no Nation* (2005), and Ishmael Beah's *A Long Way Gone: Memoirs of a Boy Soldier* (2007). Jarrett-Macauley's *Moses, Citizen and Me*, as opposed to the previously mentioned child soldier narratives, treats the rehabilitation process of child soldiers more than the underlying causes of their war trauma. It illustrates the claim that postcolonial trauma narratives tend to emphasize resilience compared to mainstream trauma narratives that often emphasize melancholia (Visser 255), showing that a "cycle of violence, wounding, and suffering" can be "broken and healed by forgiveness" (262). Failure to forgive and rehabilitate child soldiers in the aftermath of conflicts would constitute a threat of relapse into violence.

Jarrett-Macauley's *Moses, Citizen and Me* won the Orwell Prize for political writing in 2006; it deals with the rehabilitation of child soldiers who took part in the Sierra Leone Civil War (1991–2002) in which nearly 50,000 people died (Gberie 6) while countless others were physically and psychologically traumatized. It examines the effects of the Civil War on Sierra Leoneans, mainly the younger ones who are torn from their innocent childhoods to take part in the fight. Opinions differ on the fate of these children; while some of them claim their abomination and punishment for being perpetrators of violence, some others claim their forgiveness and rehabilitation for being victims of human rights crimes. In fact, international organizations like UNICEF, Human Rights Watch, Save the Children, and the Coalition to Stop the Use of Child Soldiers defend their cause, and international law protects them from being brought to trial for crimes committed during wartime under the age of 18 (Rosen 296).

The phrase "child soldier" can be read as an oxymoron. While the word "child" connotes innocence and weakness, the word "soldier" connotes agency and power. In conflict-torn regions of the world, children are usually recruited by belligerents because their lack of maturity allows better mental manipulation. Consequently, the criminal liability of abducted children is often refuted because many of them are driven to war against their will due to destitution, abandonment, or need for security when their families are decimated. From being initially represented as "dangerous and disorderly" monsters, they are now considered as "hapless victims" and sometimes "redeemed heroes" (Denov 6). Civil society organizations like Peacelinks Sierra Leone, which probably inspired Jarrett-Macauley, employed the arts to assist child soldiers in overcoming their trauma, instilling ethical values of love, peace, and nationalism through singing, dancing, drawing, acting, and other forms of artistic expression.

In *Moses, Citizen and Me*, Julia (the narrator) leaves London to visit her uncle Moses in Freetown, Sierra Leone, after the end of the Civil War. She learns that Adele, her grandmother, was killed by her grandson, George, an eight-year old "small boy" whose height is only "three feet six inches from the ground" (15). Julia observes him in the bathtub "paddling in the water with the exuberance of a duckling" and going to sleep with "the hippo brush" (46–47). Even if the community views such children as "little devils" (20), she believes her cousin is a victim; she decides to call him Citizen instead of George, saying, "Citizen, wear your name with pride. Be the country boy or be the city boy. You were never meant to be a soldier, just a *boy-citizen* first named George" (195). Even though he killed her grandmother, she understands that he was forcibly driven to do so, and she consequently forgives his action. In an article on the reintegration of child soldiers, John Williamson explains that these children are sometimes driven to kill members of their own families only to be convinced that escape is impossible; they could not return home after the horror they would have committed (189). In the studied novel, debilitating drugs and action movies are used to get hold of the children's minds, making them feel strong and commit atrocities like killing a relative.

Julia thinks about ways to let her cousin and other child soldiers return to their normal childhoods through a rehabilitative process. She visits "a care centre for children affected by the war" (31). She discovers a lifeless place with "no trees and no flowers"; the sky is "without clouds" and the sun is "hidden from view," and the ground is "solid yellow dirt with no life" with "no birds in sight" (31). In this waste land, former child soldiers queue for food; they are "not trigger-happy snipers but half-naked kids, shrieking with fear" because they have no place to call home (67). This gloomy atmosphere extends to the whole country described in the novel's opening as the land of gold and diamonds, but ravaged by internal strife. The imagery is obscure; vultures hover over the land, highlighting the pervasiveness of death while people wander with bowed heads and desperate looks.

Some former child soldiers in the novel succeed in voicing their sense of guilt, like Victor who complains that his head seems to blow up when he remembers the people he killed during the war. Another boy tries to redeem his sense of guilt by affirming that if he had not killed his victims, they would have killed him. Citizen's trauma, however, prevents him from mingling or speaking with others; when Julia attempts to break through his muteness, the only answer she can get is "no." One year after his rescue, his need to speak turns into a pathetic behavior the narrator describes in these words: "he jumped to his feet, shouting into the air, hitting and punching in a way that suggested combat with several ghostly enemies. Sounds emerged from his lips but nothing we could make sense of, no actual words – just noises and grunts that until that moment had been pinioned beneath his tongue." As if relieved from a nightmare, he keeps breathing heavily afterwards, producing "sounds of a voiceless or wild creature" (41–42). This scene highlights the claim that child soldiers shut down emotionally because they cannot cope with the burden of memory. For them, forgetting traumatic events is strenuous as these keep haunting their minds; they continually relive the past through fragmented memories, hallucinations, and nightmares. For instance, Citizen's dreams are frequently muddled by fire because he belonged to the "number-one-burning-houses unit" (53) during the war.

Scientific evidence supports that childhood trauma affects the functioning of the brain that, at this age, has not reached full maturation. Julian Ford et al. argue that children's Developmental Trauma Disorder (DTD) leads to more "extensive comorbidity" than adults' Post-traumatic stress Disorder (PTSD), associated with more "separation anxiety disorder, depression, and oppositional defiant disorder" (1). Young minds do not have the necessary coping mechanisms that allow them to deal with traumatic events, such as through speech, but their bodies keep recalling them as if they were recurring indefinitely. Hence, Bassel Van der Kolk et al. argue that rehabilitation involves the creation of "symbolic representations of past traumatic experiences, with the goals of taming the associated terror and of desomatizing the memories" (205). Since child soldiers often serve as sexual slaves, bomb carriers, or human shields, there are usually more casualties among them compared to adults. They are trained to become daredevils who do not back away from perils, but their juvenile bodies are vulnerable to debilitating drugs, sexual abuse, Sexually Transmitted Diseases, and teenage pregnancies. However, their young age gives them exceptional resilience (Klasen et al. 1096) if placed in holistic and safe environments where they engage in rehabilitative actions and interactions.

Child Soldiers' Eco-artistic Recovery

Jarrett-Macauley's *Moses, Citizen and Me* can be read through the lens of ecopsychology that analyzes the impacts of the environment on human well-being. For Theodore Roszak, the repression of the ecological unconscious is the deepest cause of malaise in modern industrial societies. He notes, "Other therapies seek to heal the alienation between person and person, person and family, person and society. Ecopsychology seeks to heal the more fundamental alienation between the person and the natural environment" (48). The "healing by nature" philosophy is regaining popularity as a way of restoring psychological and spiritual connection to the environment. In his book, *Last Child in the Woods: Saving Our Children from Nature-Deficit Disorder*, Richard Louv uses the concept of "nature-deficit disorder" to describe the negative consequences on children's minds when they have limited exposure to the natural world. Spending time in nature, he argues, enhances their cognitive abilities, increases their attention span, and enhances their well-being.

Expressive art therapy is another form of psychotherapy that facilitates nonverbal emotional expression, particularly with children who can find it difficult to express themselves verbally. The arts have liberating virtues because they make it possible to express feelings that are difficult to articulate through direct language, thus allowing the person to bypass psychic blockages. Singing, for instance, has healing potential as it tranquilizes the nerves, relieves stress, and ameliorates breathing. Dance and Movement Therapy (DMT) correspondingly facilitates interaction between dancers, permits emotional release, and prevents distressing flashbacks (Harris 207). Psychotherapists commonly use metaphors and symbols to help trauma victims express their experiences. They provide alternative frames of reference that help them remember and relate painful events without reliving the same pain. Therapeutic artistic mediation therefore makes it possible to confront the traumatic situation without re-traumatizing the victims while preventing the revival of painful memories.

Jarrett-Macauley's novel is a literary illustration of the eco-art therapy concept, also called ecological art therapy or nature-based art therapy. While the concept is new, the practice has existed since time immemorial when human beings used to live in harmony with the more-than-human world (Rust xvi). Julia's dream-like condition allows former child soldiers to be involved in eco-artistic therapy for redemptive reconstruction. To reconcile child soldiers with themselves and their community, Bemba G., the shaman, chooses a series of entertaining activities like singing, dancing, and acting to help them articulate their suffering. The idea of the healer in the forest is found in Paul Richards' *Fighting for the Rainforest* (1996); Bemba G. might be Bemba Gogbua, a storyteller "from a Gola Forest village on the Liberian border" (87). The choice of the forest is significant from an ecopsychological perspective because psychic and spiritual harmony is easier to achieve in a natural environment. It is the "place where the soul can be spoken to and re-charged, where the rational mind can let go and allow a more playful spirit in. This is not a 'cure-all' but more an offering to the imagination, a way of finding meaning in our world too full of suffering" (Rust xvi). In this sense, the artistic activities mentored by Julia and Bemba G. put the children in a situation of "eco-recovery" so that their "experience of low mood, emotional disturbance, and/or mental health treatment may be influenced by spending time out of doors, in contact with wild or domesticated animals and landscapes" (Walton 97). Significantly, Citizen spends much of his post-war time digging, and even before his abduction, his father had called him "First Citizen of the Farm" (Jarrett-Macauley 195) for his love of digging.

The forest provides a setting where the story can move back and forth between the real and the supernatural worlds, allowing healing and reintegration to happen. It is a place where the former child soldiers can be re-educated in several constructive ways imagined by Bemba G. who combines Indigenous and scientific knowledge to guide the children in their reconstruction process through deeply transformative activities. For instance, he tells of "trees that talked in the night, men who became spiders; he told forest stories that amused the eager listeners" (134). In addition to imparting moral lessons, Bemba G.'s stories provide a welcome diversion from the harsh reality of the children's former existence as soldiers; they give purpose to their lives and guidance to their futures. Research on traumatic experiences has confirmed the efficacy of storytelling as a tool for recovery; stories act as healing narratives for the psychic wounds of individuals. According to Daniel Dennett, an American philosopher, "no matter what atrocities are being narrated, the act of storytelling offers us an implicit narrative of survival to cling to, a post-trauma perspective with which to identify, and an absolute distinction between 'now' and 'then' which cordons off the narrated suffering" (418). Significantly, narrative therapy seeks to cure and empower human beings by paying greater attention to their life stories.[32] It is a therapeutic approach focused on disentangling them from their problems by externalizing their issues rather than internalizing them.

However, most human beings who have experienced trauma are usually unable to speak for themselves. This is evident in how the children freeze up when Bemba G. asks them to share their stories; he then tries other strategies to help children open up:

> Morning
> Make sure everyone eats plenty of fruit.
> Always work on mathematics first thing after breakfast.
> Games everyone can learn or join in, hide-and-seek, and dancing.
>
> Afternoon
> Playtime: work with words for Juliohs Siza!
> Child soldiers' stories.
> Rest.
> Share food.
> Sleep (don't make noise). (Jarrett-Macauley 144)

The mathematics activity is intended to enhance children's logical reasoning, keeping them occupied and quiet while reawakening their curiosity about the pleasant realm of numbers, abstract thinking and problem-solving. Bemba G. involves them in the "HA" game, and as soon as he utters the word "Ha," laughter ensues among the children. Instantaneously, their spirits lift, marked by joyous shouts and leaps (135). The children ultimately dance in a kind of trance, singing, "If you're happy and you know it, clap your hands" (202). These are signs of resilience that herald a potentially recoverable innocence and peace.

Perhaps the most important activity is the one in which the children act in an adaptation of William Shakespeare's *Julius Caesar* entitled *Juliohs Siza* (1964), written in the local language by the Sierra Leonean playwright Thomas Decker. By translating this play, Decker warns his people against the perils of absolute power. In addition to appropriating the potent political message that *Julius Caesar* might convey to a newly independent nation, Tcho Mbaimba Caulker argues that Decker's translation is probably "an attempt to deliver an important political message to the new nation on the subject of governance through the example and representation of a once noble servant of the Roman people turned hubristic emperor" (209). The message to Sierra Leoneans might not only be a praise of democracy, but also a warning on the possible outcomes in case of diversion from it (212–213).

---

32 See Michael White and David Epston's *Narrative Means to Therapeutic Ends*. W. W. Norton, 1990.

In Jarrett-Macauley's novel, the children are initially gripped by performance anxiety. Bemba G. explains that this feeling is different from the fear they used to have during the war (177), and he gives them "a rainforest drink" (177) to let them feel "strong" and "courageous" (178). At this stage, "Real fear is being converted into fictional fear" (Müller-Thalheim 166), and it can be more easily confronted and articulated. Miriam, who plays the role of Portia, represents little girl soldiers; she has a nameless baby conceived in a gang rape. She bravely perplexes the audience by taking off her gown to show the lacerations that cover her body, indelible proofs of the torture inflicted on her during the Civil War. As part of her therapy, Miriam shocks her audience to make them aware of the horrors endured by innocents.

The children gradually acquire self-confidence, communication, and collaboration skills through acting. When Citizen cannot speak, another child interpolates, "We must not press Citizen to say 'yes' if he wants time to think" (Jarrett-Macauley 179). The children argue that it would be sufficient if he preferred to sing instead, highlighting their understanding of the democratic lessons of the play. Citizen sings in a "flute voice" that fills the listeners' ears (206), and Julia, who has been waiting for the time he could speak again, enjoys his performance; it is, for her, an enormous act of courage (186). Singing in the play is "cathartic"; it allows "Citizen to finally leave the past behind" (Whitehead 255–256). A crucial moment in his rehabilitation happens in the middle of the play. When he sleeps and dreams of his grandmother absolving him and praying for him, his face speaks "of a heart softening from fossil to pearly shell" that is "ready to be broken"; he eventually "thinks of tenderness and love – joining hands" (Jarrett-Macauley 207–208). With his grandmother's prayer, his hands let go of the gun as the murderous spell vanishes.

For Julia, acting allows the "ending of amnesia" because the children find "themselves in the play" and "their place in the scheme of things" (159). By acting their roles in the play, child soldiers can sense the causes of their trauma, like political rivalry and family violence, for which they are not guilty. The performance ends with the children's choral song, a moment of music therapy in front of an international audience whose voice is attuned to theirs: "Peace, Freedom, Liberty! Peace, Freedom, Liberty!" (205). The audience is "a mixed bunch, a medley of ages, nationalities and types: British and American soldiers in uniform, village people from across the river, some of the Freetown elites with their own kerosene lamps in hand, and more child soldiers walking barefoot" (201). The diversity of the audience symbolizes the need to involve diverse stakeholders in the rehabilitation of former child soldiers.

Child Soldiers' Rite of Passage in the Archetypal Forest

In *From Ritual to Theatre: The Human Seriousness of Play,* Victor Turner considers "social dramas" as a way of addressing issues and highlighting solutions in an indirect manner. He considers drama as a major element of the "redressive machinery" whose purpose is "to patch up quarrels, 'mend' broken social ties, 'seal up punctures' in the 'social fabric'" (10). Neophytes, child soldiers in *Moses, Citizen and Me,* are dislocated from their sociocultural structure and thrown into a liminal situation in which they "are betwixt and between the positions assigned and arrayed by law, custom, convention, and ceremonial" (*Ritual Process* 95). Their rite of passage through drama ends with their reincorporation into the sociocultural structure and the acquisition of knowledge that alters their innermost beings, giving them a better status within the community. Liminality in the forest brings about benefits for the children, as it creates a change from "I to Thou," a longing for "communitas," the Latin term that Turner distinguishes from "community." In his view, "communitas" involves a feeling of intimacy between individuals who go through liminality as a group (359–360). In this state of "communitas," a distinctive sense of intimacy emerges among individuals who go through the liminal journey as a group; by strengthening their bonds, a sense of unity emerges, creating a powerful collective identity. This experience gives a gift of knowledge, a humanistic conscience, and an ability to create lasting bonds that help in the healing process of the former child soldiers.

In a symbolic action towards healing, Citizen carves "439K" into a wooden block; it is the numerical soldier identity "cut into his back." He buries the curved number while Julia comments:

> Citizen, lingering behind me, looked relieved, as though he had given up a world. The block of wood rested on the mat before me. I could barely keep my eyes off it, so assertive was its presence. Citizen had needed to make it and I had needed to see it. [...] I began with a wish for the future: that the 439K scar would not follow him to his grave, that Citizen be free of 439K. [...] "Let's bury this," I suggested, "let's lay it to rest." He agreed. (Jarrett-Macauley 164)

After burying the wooden block, Citizen feels "rested" like "a freshly washed child" (165–166); he is on his path of healing. This longing for attention and affection was initially symbolized by his small hands, and as he gradually feels better, his hands grow larger: "Kindness had slipped into his body like heartsease, permitting his hands to grow. Over the next few weeks, changing like molten glass forged in fire, Citizen's hand grew big. Forgiveness came" (219). The growing hands symbolically coincide with the coming of the journalist to whom Citizen recounts his grandmother's murder; his trauma is finally finding its way towards articulation.

His growing hands "circle the air in rapid motion" like "a ruddy brown butterfly boy" (161); the dumb, motionless boy happily turns into a flying creature.

Just like the traumatized children, Moses, Julia's uncle and Citizen's grandfather, is initially incapable of voicing his trauma. He confides to Julia, "Don't know how I can begin to tell you" (11); not until the end of the novel could he recount the circumstances in which his wife was murdered. He, too, finds a therapeutic outlet through art. He creates a photographic archive of famous West African photographers like Alphonso Lisk-Carew and John Parkes Decker, as well as his own. He finds refuge in "his memories, understanding the pleasure to be gained from squeezing oneself back in time and space" (43). He enjoys stepping back into a peaceful time, "a world away from the chaotic Freetown" of his day. The reality is sad, but in those photographs, there is "no sign of despair, death, war and mutilation" (44). Julia observes the photographs of Citizen before the Civil War, "at every stage of his young life" (98); she commiserates the loss of his parents and his innocence. She tries to reconcile Moses and Citizen, initially each with himself, and eventually with each other; "the family narrative thus comes to stand as a microcosm for the broader social difficulty of post-war reconciliation in Sierra Leone" (Whitehead 242). Moses permits Citizen to return home from the sylvan rehabilitation camp while many "people will not even let a child like Citizen near their house after what he's done. They cannot stand the sight of them. They believe they are little devils" (Jarrett-Macauley 19–20). The eco-artistic rehabilitation initiative not only heals the former child soldiers, but also their community, allowing each one to forgive and move forward.

By the end of the novel, the children are driven to be whole again; they are indeed driven to feel human after the bestial actions they were compelled to perform. They collectively read an empowering poem: *"Dear child / You feel the flow of blood in your veins / The beat of your heart / You are powerful, indeed"* (151). The children receive support from nature as they recover; the sky is clear, and they all take a long stroll to the stream where they swim and play along the water's edge. This flowing stream at the end of the novel represents their transformation from children who are stuck in the traumatic past to ones that move forward peacefully. In a way that atones for the sins committed against the land, the rain pours down to cleanse it. The children step out into the blue haze and stroll back while the sun shines more brilliantly than ever before (186–187). Because they witnessed death at an early age, the cycle of nature can teach them existential lessons on impermanence and regeneration. During their eco-artistic activities, nature serves as a facilitator of their healing journey. They observe and interact with the natural world, seeking inspiration, guidance, and solace; they engage in sensory experiences to deepen the connection with natural elements, like touching the texture of the soil, smelling plants, listening to nature sounds, and contemplating the colors and shapes around them. This mindful sensory engagement can reduce toxic stress, evoke positive emotions, induce useful self-awareness, and enhance much-needed well-being.

Conclusion

Jarret-Macaulay's *Moses, Citizen and Me* is a valuable resource for learning about the suffering of child soldiers and the trauma that war brings onto their minds. The novel offers an illustration of therapeutic artistic mediation that takes charge of child soldiers in a holistic approach; it also shows a vision of communitas that serves as group therapy. The forest where the children have served as soldiers turns into a healing place where they are rehabilitated via eco-artistic ritualization. Expressive art therapy offers them a non-verbal means to safely channel their feelings through symbolic representations that create a safe distance from the experienced trauma. In this setting, they can conjure up memories and emotions that might otherwise be challenging to articulate verbally. Because the arts encourage self-expression, they allow child soldiers to reconnect with their inner selves and explore their personal narratives.

Conclusion

Devoted to the inclusive ambition of global health humanities, this book journeyed through the global Anglophone literary world in search of novels that answer global health issues, pausing at significant milestones with African American, British-Indian, British-Sierra Leonean, Indian, Kenyan, Native American, Pakistani, Trinidadian-Canadian, South African, South African-Australian, and Zimbabwean authors. The adopted global health humanities approach reimagined healthcare in a holistic, equitable, and compassionate manner, addressing not only the physical but also the mental, emotional, and social aspects of health and well-being. Embracing the "One Health" approach, it also assigned equal importance to humans and more-than-humans. The green dimension of this book, or global environmental health humanities, highlights the therapeutic influence of nature, the invaluable contribution of biodiversity to medicine, and the psychological relief offered by natural landscapes. The culturally diverse global Anglophone novels studied in it advocate for global equity, sustainable living, and holistic healthcare.

The first part of this book mapped the terrain of global health humanities in relation to literature by prompting readers into an interdisciplinary exploration of the blossoming field. The aim was to emphasize the role of the global Anglophone novel in comprehending the relationship between global health and human experience, with related historical, sociocultural, and ethical implications. By calling attention to the intersectional aspects of health, disease, and disability, in relation to race, gender, and class, this part indicated the contribution of global health humanities, including the global Anglophone novel, in enhancing a more inclusive and equitable healthcare. In so doing, it laid the foundation for the following parts to illustrate the concept of applied literature on disease and disability across a wide geographical span.

Integrating postcolonial theory into global health humanities allowed for a close reading wherein marginalized voices subvert dominant narratives that perpetuate inequalities in the field of health. Clearly, colonization has left indelible imprints on the psyche of the colonized as it has induced nervous conditions that plague the colonized, decades after the independence of their nations. The book highlighted the importance of considering Fanon's contributions to global health humanities with his socioculturally sensitive approach to mental health treatment, challenging the discourse of colonial psychiatry that ignored the sociocultural dimensions of mental health. He believes that even more destructive than the colonization of the land is the colonization of the mind, requiring not just political independence, but also psychological independence. This objective requires the subversion of master narratives that have perpetuated stereotypes about the colonized body as diseased, disabled, repulsive, or monstrous.

Using the postcolonial theory, this book questioned the presence of a unique knowledge system, as it involved the recognition of diverse ways of knowing the world. It promoted a more inclusive academic landscape by opening up spaces for marginalized voices to understand the challenges of global health. Exploring the postcolonial perspective on trauma was useful to consider the suffering of marginalized communities around the world, contesting dominant narratives, dismantling stereotypes, and promoting social equity. It also highlighted the psychological impact of cultural displacement and estrangement in the context of migration, as well as the psychological toll of gender-based violence.

The second part of this book focused on infectious diseases, like smallpox, cholera, malaria, and AIDS to bring out the effect of epidemics on diverse human behaviors and societal responses, mainly in the context of health inequalities. Special attention was given to the role of global flows in the spread of epidemics, starting with imperial expansion to globalization. It reflected on virgin soil epidemics and unresolved traumatic grief in Erdrich's *Tracks*, as well as Indigenous healing traditions used to mend wounds, foster resilience, and ensure survivance. This part likewise explored the colonial history of epidemiology in Ghosh's *The Calcutta Chromosome: A Novel of Fevers, Delirium, and Discovery* that attributes the discovery of the malaria parasite to a secret Indian medical group instead of the British physician Robert Ross. The author uses the metaphor of the chromosome to represent the complementarity of Euro-America-centric and Indigenous knowledge systems, emphasizing the need to embrace their harmonious blend for a comprehensive understanding of health. This part finally analyzed Mwangi's criticism of behaviors that contribute to the spread of HIV/AIDS such as wife inheritance, multiple sexual partnerships, and resistance to condoms in *Crossroads: The Last Plague*. He also illustrates the power of "Accelerated Inner Development Syndrome" in transforming corporeal deterioration into soul restoration, providing graceful acceptance of the ebbs and flows of life.

The third part of the book examined the portrayal of mental disorders, like bulimia, anorexia nervosa, depression, trauma, schizophrenia, and dementia to explore the effects of slavery, colonialism, and migration on psychic health. It explored the lives and minds of American characters from different ethnicities in Morrison's *A Mercy* to understand their struggle with the trauma of maternal abandonment. Mothers who faced the sorrowful choice to forsake their children, the author shows, did so out of the intent to shield them from the horrors of slavery. This part also penetrated the lives and minds of Zimbabwean females in Dangarembga's trilogy to comprehend the patriarchal and colonial roots of their nervous conditions like eating disorders and depression. It finally studied the topic of presenile dementia in Chariandy's *Soucouyant*, in relation to life fragmentation, immigrant subjectivity, and multicultural assimilation in Canada.

The fourth part of the book researched the world of disability to go beyond its interpretation as a metaphor or "narrative prosthesis" (Mitchell and Snyder 49) in literary works. Although it is actually represented as such in some selected novels, an empathic reading allowed a more realistic interpretation. It showed, for instance, that Sidhwa's *Cracking India* relies on the metaphor of the disabled body to represent the fractured social structure of the Indian subcontinent after the Partition, hence illustrating Mitchell and Snyder's concept of "narrative prosthesis." However, the novel lends itself to other readings using Quayson's concept of "aesthetic nervousness" and typology of disability representation. This part equally highlighted that Rushdie's *Shame* pushes the metaphoric representations of disability and ableist attitudes to a magical realist extreme by equating the experience of disability with shame and monstrosity in a Pakistani setting. Yet, an empathic reading uncovers the humanity of the autistic character and the opprobrium rebounds on the ableist society, challenging readers to face their own biases and to reflect on a more empathic and inclusive society. Finally, this part showed that Coetzee's *Slow Man* criticizes the paternalistic "doctor-patient" model in an Australian healthcare setting, emphasizing the need for a therapeutic alliance centered on the care seeker's humanity and active role in the healing journey. It invites readers to reflect on their social conceptions of disability, aging, and caregiving. The experience might provoke a sense of discomfort that, in turn, urges readers to question their own ableist attitudes.

The last part of the book on holistic healing rekindled attention to ethnomedical practices that can contribute, in conjunction with biomedical practices, to the health and well-being of human beings. It equally celebrated the role of nature in holistic healing approaches like forest therapy, garden therapy, and eco-artistic recovery. It brought the book to a closure by showing the importance of the green dimension to global health humanities. This concert takes humans back to the primeval times when art was not only a means of creative expression, but also a ritualistic performance in the natural environment to solicit the forces of nature for nourishment and protection. The remembrance draws attention to the need for a holistic and sustainable perspective on global health challenges. This part studied the power of autopathography in Head's *A Question of Power*, disclosing the sociohistorical etiology of insanity in an apartheid South African setting, as well as the healing potential of communal gardening with its spiritual and transcendental dimensions. It likewise demonstrated the redemptive power of storytelling and environmentalism in Silko's *Ceremony*, illustrating the importance of restoring the broken bond with the land and the community to heal the protagonist's intergenerational trauma and Post-Traumatic Stress Disorder. It finally provided an instance of therapeutic artistic mediation in the rehabilitation of Sierra Leonean child soldiers through the literary analysis of Jarrett-Macauley's *Moses, Citizen and Me*. Ultimately, the forest where they served as soldiers turns into a place of eco-artistic ritualization.

Reading the selected novels eventually substantiated the view that the division of the book into five parts was just a response to structural necessities while in reality, the five parts overlapped considerably. For instance, some infectious diseases have an impact on mental health, causing anxiety, depression, and trauma while other infectious diseases can cause long-term disabilities. Mental disorders can lead to disability and disability can have a toll on mental health. Ultimately, in all cases of health and unhealth, human beings require holistic interventions where the natural environment plays a pivotal role.

By applying global health humanities to the global Anglophone novel, this book demonstrated that healthcare is not solely a matter of biomedical understanding, but is in like manner, a matter of historical legacies, social structures, and cultural practices. It also evinced that biomedicine is not the sole approach to disease and disability, and that it can benefit from consolidation with ethnomedicine. While the selected novels place significant stress on holistic healing practices, rooted in nature and culture, their reading also underlines that the status of biomedicine remains unquestionable. Reading the selected global Anglophone novels illustrated the complementary nature of biomedicine and ethnomedicine, advocating for their integration to cultivate a global health humanities approach centered on the care seeker. While biomedicine excels in empirical diagnosis and treatment, the novelists exemplify, ethnomedicine drives home the holistic healing principles that consider various dimensions of health. Their affirmation of therapeutic alliance exemplifies the departure from paternalistic to collaborative relationships between the care provider and the care seeker. Their culturally competent healing solutions appreciate the influence of cultural lore in enhancing inclusivity and reducing inequality. By incorporating nature into narrative, the selected global Anglophone novels promote a holistic healing approach that involves the physical, emotional, and spiritual well-being of the care seeker.

With forethought, this book integrated the following Sustainable Development Goals (SDGs) through the literary analysis of global Anglophone novels:

– Good Health and Well-being (SDG 3): It analyzed physical and mental health, sociocultural determinants of health, therapeutic storytelling, creative arts therapy, etc.
– Quality Education (SDG 4): It stressed the transformative potential of literature and the humanities in healthcare education, promoting critical thinking, diversity, and inclusion.

- Gender Equality (SDG 5): It illustrated the effects of patriarchal systems and gender-based violence on female health.
- Reduced Inequalities (SDG 10): It underlined healthcare disparities between the Global South and the Global North, as well between different ethnic groups in the Global North.
- Life on land (SDG 15): It dealt with the topics of environmental injustice, environmental activism, garden therapy, and eco-artistic recovery.
- Peace, justice, and strong institutions (SDG 16): It explored the effects of slavery, colonialism, globalization, and migration on health.
- Partnerships for the Goals (SDG 17): It highlighted the importance of global methodology in teaching and research.

The preceding list shows that Literature plays a role in advancing the Sustainable Development Goals by fostering awareness, empathy, and critical thinking. Making complex issues accessible to a wide audience, it serves as a vehicle for advocating social justice and environmental stewardship. Consequently, it is useful to consider the role of global Anglophone literature in advancing the United Nations' Sustainable Development Goals, mainly Good Health and Wellbeing, giving center stage to marginalized voices in the field of global health.

As befits a book with an interdisciplinary aspiration, it is important de consider the pedagogical implications of teaching the global Anglophone novel in the field of global health humanities to foster "flexibility, adaptability, creativity, cultural sensitivity, and cross-cultural communication skills" (Stewart and Swain 2586). One of the potential implications of reading global Anglophone novels on disease, disability, health, and well-being is to provide a platform for the exploration of diverse cultural reactions to them, allowing students to develop cultural awareness and to appreciate the specificities of different societies. Through this imaginary exposure, they become more attuned to the cultural contexts they may encounter in global health settings. Another potential implication of teaching the global Anglophone novel in the field of global health humanities is to hone students' critical thinking and analytical skills by analyzing characters, themes, and metaphors with ethical import to global health. This imaginary exposure enhances projection and empathy, two necessary qualities for compassionate healthcare. It is also likely to foster cross-cultural communication, much needed by global health professionals who essentially work in foreign settings, through the study of interactions between characters from various cultural backgrounds in imaginary situations related to disease, disability, health, and well-being. Exposure to such novels leads students to venture beyond established paradigms because literature stimulates imagination and creativity; this skill is essential in the field of global health where singular challenges demand constant reflection. The inclusivity of this approach eventually allows students to visit unfamiliar situations with the resourcefulness acquired through the vicarious experience of reading.

As much remains to be written in this growing field of global health humanities, more intersectional studies are useful to explore the effects of race, gender, and class on the subjectivity of diseased and disabled corporeality. Another beneficial avenue of research will be the exploration of global Anglophone novels through the lens of narrative medicine and ethics of care to enhance empathy, communication, and interconnectedness between healthcare providers, caregivers, and care seekers. Addressing these topics through a comparative approach would be challenging, but it would highlight similarities and differences in health and healthcare in a mosaic of diverse cultures. The vision is of a future where more empathic and equitable healthcare systems thrive, encompassing not just the mending of bodies but also the uplifting of spirits. In this future, reading literature from diverse cultural backgrounds will cultivate feelings of empathy and shared humanity. In a very recent article entitled "Health humanities for inclusive, globally interdependent, supportive and decolonised health professional education: The future is health humanities!" Sandra E. Carr & Claire Hooker believe that this field promises "imaginative and joyful innovations" in health professions education in the forthcoming 50 years (123). The future is, as I see it, in global environmental health humanities.

Works Cited

Abdel-Halim, Rabie E. "The Role of Ibn Sina (Avicenna)'s Medical Poem in the Transmission of Medical Knowledge to Medieval Europe." *Urology Annals*, vol. 6, no. 1, 2014, pp. 1–12. www.ncbi.nlm.nih.gov/pmc/articles/PMC3963335/pdf/UA-6-1.pdf. Accessed 30 Nov. 2022.

Achenbaum, W. Andrew. *Robert Butler MD: Visionary of Healthy Aging*. Columbia University Press, 2013.

Affun-Adegbulu, Clara, and Adegbulu Opemiposi. "Decolonising Global (Public) Health: From Western Universalism to Global Pluriversalities." *BMJ Global Health*, vol. 5, no. 8, 2020, pp. 1–3. www.gh.bmj.com/content/bmjgh/5/8/e002947.full.pdf. Accessed 5 Sep. 2022.

Allen, Paula G. "The Sacred Hoop." *The Ecocriticism Reader: Landmarks in Literary Ecology*, edited by Cheryll Glotfelty and Harold Fromm. Georgia University Press, 1996, pp. 241–263.

Allen, Paula G. *The Sacred Hoop: Recovering the Feminine in American Indian Traditions*. Beacon Press, 1986.

American Veterinary Medical Association. "One Health: A New Professional Imperative." 15 Jul. 2008. www.avma.org/sites/default/files/resources/onehealth_final.pdf. Accessed 2 Nov. 2023.

Anderson, Warwick. *The Cultivation of Whiteness: Science, Health and Racial Destiny in Australia*. Melbourne University Press, 2003.

Anderson, Warwick. "Where is the Postcolonial History of Medicine?" *Bulletin of the History of Medicine*, no. 72, 1998, pp. 522–530. www.pubmed.ncbi.nlm.nih.gov/9780451/. Accessed 10 Apr. 2023.

Apte, C. Vasudha. "History of Medicine: Sir Ronald Ross (Born 13 May 1857, died 16 Sep 1932)." *Medical Journal Armed Forces India*, vol. 53, no. 1, 1997, pp. 68–69. www.ncbi.nlm.nih.gov/pmc/articles/PMC5530821/. Accessed 17 Nov. 2022.

Ashcroft, Bill, et al. "The Body and Performance." *The Postcolonial Studies Reader*, edited by Bill Ashcroft, et al. Routledge, 1995, pp. 321–322.

Ashcroft, Bill, et al. *The Empire Writes Back: Theory and Practice in Post-Colonial Literatures*. Routledge, 1989.

Bachner-Melman, Rachel, and Beth A. Oakley. "Giving 'Till it Hurts': Eating Disorders and Pathological Altruism." *Bio-Psycho-Social Contributions to Understanding Eating Disorders*, edited by Yael Latzer and Daniel Stein. Springer, 2016, pp. 91–103.

Barker, Clare. *Postcolonial Fiction and Disability: Exceptional Children, Metaphor and Materiality*. Palgrave Macmillan, 2011.

Bastian, Dawn, and Judy Mitchell. *Handbook of Native American Mythology*. ABC-CLIO, 2004.

Battiste, Marie. "Indigenous Knowledge: Foundations for First Nations." *WINHEC: International Journal of Indigenous Education Scholarship*, no. 1, pp. 1–12. www.journals.uvic.ca/index.php/winhec/article/view/19251. Accessed 12 Feb. 2023.

Beard, Linda S. "Bessie Head in Gaborone, Botswana: An Interview." *Sage*, vol. 3, no. 2, 1986, pp. 44–47.

Benatar, Solomon. "Politics, Power, Poverty and Global Health: Systems and Frames." *International Journal of Health Policy and Management*, no, 5, 2016, pp. 599–604. www.ncbi.nlm.nih.gov/pmc/articles/PMC5042589/. Accessed 2 Oct. 2023.

Betancourt, Joseph R., et al. "Defining Cultural Competence: A Practical Framework for Addressing Racial/Ethnic Disparities in Health and Health Care." *Public Health Reports*, vol. 118, no. 4, 2003, pp. 293–302. www.ncbi.nlm.nih.gov/pmc/articles/PMC1497553/pdf/12815076.pdf. Accessed 10 Oct. 2022.

Bleakley, Alan, et al. "Thinking the Post-colonial in Medical Education." *Medical Education*, vol. 42, no. 3, 2008, pp. 266–270. www.pubmed.ncbi.nlm.nih.gov/18275413/. Accessed 8 Jan. 2023.

Boehmer, Elleke. *Stories of Women: Gender and Narrative in the Postcolonial Nation*. Manchester University Press, 2005.

Bowlby, John. *Child Care and the Growth of Love*. Pelican Book, 1972.

Brandt, Allan M. "Racism and Research: The Case of the Tuskegee Syphilis Study." *The Hastings Center Report*, vol. 8, no. 6, 1978, pp. 21–29. www.dash.harvard.edu/bitstream/handle/1/3372911/Brandt_Racism.pdf?isAllowed=y&sequence=1. Accessed 10 Nov. 2022.

Brave Heart, Maria Y. H. "The Historical Trauma Response among Natives and its Relationship with Substance Abuse: A Lakota Illustration." *Journal of Psychoactive Drugs*, vol. 35, no. 1, 2003, pp. 7–13. www.pubmed.ncbi.nlm.nih.gov/12733753/. Accessed 9 Feb. 2023.

Brave Heart, Maria Y. H., and Lemyra M. DeBruyn. "The American Indian Holocaust: Healing Historical Unresolved Grief." *American Indian and Alaska Native Mental Health Research*, vol. 8, no. 2, 1998, pp. 60–82. www.proquest.com/docview/236003962. Accessed 9 Feb. 2023.

Brison, Susan J. "Trauma Narratives and the Remaking of the Self." *Acts of Memory: Cultural Recall in the Present*, edited by Mieke Bal, et al. Dartmouth College, 1999, pp. 39–54.

Brody, Howard. "Defining the Medical Humanities: Three Conceptions and Three Narratives." *Journal of Medical Humanities*, vol. 32, no. 1, 2011, pp. 1–7. www.pubmed.ncbi.nlm.nih.gov/19936898/. Accessed 11 Nov. 2022.

Brumberg, Joan J. *Fasting Girls: The Emergence of Anorexia Nervosa as a Modern Disease*. Harvard University Press, 1988.

Burns, Paul, and Richard McKane. "Metaphor and Trauma: Poetry from Clean Language Questions." *Fulcrum: An Annual of Poetry and Aesthetics*, vol. 3, 2004, pp. 303–316.

Butler, Judith. *Frames of War: When is Life Grievable?* Verso, 2009.

Butler, Robert N. "Appendix: Prologue or Introduction to Life Review." 2010. *Robert Butler MD: Visionary of Healthy Aging*, edited by W. Andrew Achenbaum. Columbia University Press, 2013, pp. 199–218.

Calvino, Italo. *Six Memos for the Next Millennium*. Translated by Patrick Creagh, Vintage, 1996.

Campbell, Fiona K. *Contours of Ableism: The Production of Disability and Abledness*. Palgrave Macmillan, 2009.

Caracciolo, Marco. "Patterns of Cognitive Dissonance in Readers' Engagement with Characters." *Enthymema*, no. 8, 2013, pp. 21–37. www.pure.rug.nl/ws/portalfiles/portal/55378780/document.pdf. Accessed 14 Dec. 2023.

Carr, Sandra E., and Hooker, Claire. "Health Humanities for Inclusive, Globally Interdependent, Supportive and Decolonised Health Professional Education: The Future Is Health Humanities!" *Focus On Health Professional Education*, vol. 24, no. 4, 2023, pp. 123–135. www.fohpe.org/FoHPE/article/view/721/382. Accessed 27 Jan. 2024.

Caruth, Cathy. *Trauma: Explorations in Memory*. Johns Hopkins University Press, 1995.

Caulker, Tcho M. "Shakespeare's *Julius Caesar* in Sierra Leone: Thomas Decker's *Juliohs Siza*, Roman Politics, and the Emergence of a Postcolonial African State." *Research in African Literatures*, vol. 4, no. 2, 2009, pp. 208–227. www.muse.jhu.edu/journals/research_in_african_literatures/v040/40.2.caulker.pdf. Accessed 1 Feb. 2023.

CDC. "Ross and the Discovery that Mosquitoes Transmit Malaria Parasites," 2015. www.cdc.gov/malaria/about/history/ross.html. Accessed 5 Jan. 2023.

Chambers, Claire. "Networks of Stories: Amitav Ghosh's *The Calcutta Chromosome*". *Ariel*, vol. 40, no. 2–3, 2009, pp. 41–62. www.journalhosting.ucalgary.ca/index.php/ariel/article/view/34892/28910. Accessed 12 Jul. 2022.

Chariandy, David. "David Chariandy: 'To Make Sense of Prejudice, Tell the Story of the Past." Interview with Kate Kellaway. *The Guardian*, 14 Apr. 2019. www.theguardian.com/books/2019/apr/14/david-chariandy-ive-been-meaning-to-tell-you-father-advice-to-daughter. Accessed 10 Jan. 2021.

Chariandy, David. *I've Been Meaning to Tell you: A Letter to my Daughter*. Bloomsbury, 2018.

Chariandy, David. *Soucouyant*. Arsenal Pulp Press, 2007.

Chariandy, David. "Spirits of Elsewhere Past: A Dialogue on *Soucouyant*." Interview with Kit Dobson. *Callaloo*, vol. 30, no. 3, 2007, pp. 808–817. www.jstor.org/stable/30139278. Accessed 10 Jan. 2021.

Charon, Rita, et al. "Literature and Medicine: Contributions to Clinical Practice." *Annals of Internal Medicine*, vol. 122, no. 8, 1995, pp. 599–606. www.pubmed.ncbi.nlm.nih.gov/7887555/. Accessed 18 Nov. 2020.

Charon, Rita. "Close Reading: The Signature Method of Narrative Medicine." *The Principles and Practice of Narrative Medicine*, edited by Rita Charon, et al. Oxford Academic, 2016, pp. 157–179.

Coetzee, John M. *Slow Man*, Martin Secker & Warburg, 2005.

Cole, Teju. "Unmournable Bodies." *The New Yorker*, 9 Jan. 2015, pp. 1–5. www.newyorker.com/culture/cultural-comment/unmournable-bodies. Accessed 10 Jul. 2019.

Cole, Thomas R., et al. *Medical Humanities: An Introduction*. Cambridge University Press, 2015.

Couser, G. Thomas. "Disability, Life Narrative, and Representation." *The Disability Studies Reader*, edited by Lennard J. Davis. Routledge, 2013, pp. 456–459.

Craps, Stef. *Postcolonial Witnessing: Trauma Out of Bonds*. Palgrave Macmillan, 2013.

Craps, Stef. "Wor(l)ds of Grief: Traumatic Memory and Literary Witnessing in Cross-Cultural Perspective." *Textual Practice*, vol. 24, no. 1, 2010, pp. 51–68. www.tandfonline.com/doi/abs/10.1080/09502360903219808. Accessed 10 Apr. 2015.

Crawford, Allison, et al. "Indigenous Health Humanities." *The Routledge Companion to Health Humanities*, edited by Paul Crawford, et al. Routledge, 2020, pp. 96–105.

Crawford, Paul, et al. "Applied Literature." *Health Humanities*. Palgrave Macmillan, 2015, pp. 38–59.

Crawford, Paul, et al. "Health Humanities: The Future of Medical Humanities?" *Mental Health Review Journal*, vol. 15, no. 3, 2010, pp. 4–10. www.emerald.com/insight/content/doi/10.5042/mhrj.2010.0654/full/html. Accessed 20 Apr. 2022.

Crawford, Paul. "Introduction: Global Health Humanities and the Rise of Creative Public Health." *The Routledge Companion to Health Humanities*, edited by Paul Crawford, et al. Routledge, 2020, pp. 1–7.

Crosby, Alfred W. *Ecological Imperialism: The Biological Expansion of Europe*. Cambridge University Press, 1986.

Crosby, Alfred W. "Virgin Soil Epidemics as a Factor in the Aboriginal Depopulation in America." *The William and Mary Quarterly*, vol. 33, no. 2, 1976, pp. 289–299. www.sjsu.edu/people/ruma.chopra/courses/H210a_S13/s0/B_Crosby_VirSoilEpid.pdf Accessed 17 Mar. 2021.

Cuddon, John A. *The Penguin Dictionary of Literary Terms and Literary Theory*. 1976. Revised ed. by Claire E. Preston, Penguin Books, 1998.

Cunsolo, Ashlee, and Neville R. Ellis. "Ecological Grief as a Mental Health Response to Climate Change-related Loss." *Nature Climate Change*, vol. 8, no. 4, 2018, pp. 275–281. www.nature.com/articles/s41558-018-0092-2. Accessed 12 Jan. 2020.

Dangarembga, Tsitsi. *The Book of Not.* Faber, 2006.
Dangarembga, Tsitsi. *This Mournable Body.* Graywolf Press, 2018.
Dangarembga, Tsitsi. *Nervous Conditions.* Zimbabwe Publishing House, 1988.
Darian-Smith, Eve, and Philip C. McCarthy. *The Global Turn: Theories, Research Designs, and Methods for Global Studies.* University of California Press, 2017.
DasGupta, Sayantani. "Visionary Medicine: Race, Health, Power, and Speculation" *The Routledge Companion to Health Humanities*, edited by Paul Crawford, et al. Routledge, 2020, pp. 33–38.
Davis, Lennard J. "Constructing Normalcy: The Bell Curve, the Novel, and the Invention of the Disabled Body in the Nineteenth Century." *The Disability Studies Reader*, edited by Lennard J. Davis, 2nd ed. Routledge, 2006, pp. 3–16.
Davis, Lennard J. "Crips Strike Back: The Rise of Disability Studies." *American Literary History*, vol. 11, no. 3, 1999, pp. 500–512. www.jstor.org/stable/490130. Accessed 12 Jul. 2022.
Dennett, Daniel. *Consciousness Explained.* Allen Lane/Penguin Press, 1991.
Denov, Myriam. *Child Soldiers: Sierra Leone's Revolutionary United Front.* Cambridge University Press, 2010.
Derrida, Jacque. *Psyche: Inventions of the Other*, vol. 1, edited by Peggy Kamuf & Elizabeth Rottenberg. Stanford University Press, 2007.
Dudley, Rachel. "The Role of Feminist Health Humanities Scholarship and Black Women's Artistry in Re-Shaping the Origin Narrative of Modern, U.S. Gynecology." *Humanities*, vol. 10, no. 1, 2021, pp. 1–18. www.mdpi.com/2076–0787/10/1/58. Accessed 18 Nov. 2022.
Dyson, Tim. *A Population History of India: From the First Modern People to the Present Day.* Oxford University Press, 2018.
Edwards, Justin D. " 'She Saw a Soucouyant': Locating the Globalgothic." *Globalgothic*, edited by Glennis Byron. Manchester University Press, 2013, pp. 50–64.
Eklöf Amirell, Stefan. "From Global Studies to Global Humanities." Humanities, vol. 12, no. 2, 2023, pp. 1–14. www.diva-portal.org/smash/get/diva2:1759765/FULLTEXT01.pdf. Accessed 1 Dec. 2023.
El-Hadi, Nehal. "The Palimpsest: Black and Ethnic Minority Perspectives in Health Humanities." *The Routledge Companion to Health Humanities*, edited by Paul Crawford, et al. Routledge, 2020, pp. 43–48.
Eliade, Mircea. *Myth and Reality.* Translated by Willard R. Trask. Harper & Row, 1963.
Engel, George L. "The Need for a New Medical Model: A Challenge for Biomedicine." *Science*, vol. 196, no. 4286, 1977, pp. 129–136. www.pubmed.ncbi.nlm.nih.gov/847460/. Accessed 20 Nov. 2023.
Erdrich, Louise. *Tracks.* Henry Holt, 1988.
"Etymological Explorations and the Choreography of Trauma." Ebrary.net. www.ebrary.net/142526/sociology/etymological_explorations_choreography_trauma. Accessed 15 Oct. 2022.
Fahey, Joseph, and Richard Armstrong. *A Peace Reader: Essential Readings on War, Justice, Non-violence and World Order.* Paulist Press International, 1992.
Falco, Elena. "The Convoluted History of the Double Helix." The Royal Society, 2018. www.royalsociety.org/blog/2018/04/history-of-the-double-helix/. Accessed 3 Jun. 2023.
Fanon, Frantz. *Black Skin, White Masks.* 1952. Translated by Richard Philcox, Grove Press, 2008.
Fanon, Frantz. *A Dying Colonialism.* 1959. Translated by Henri Chevalier, Grove Press, 1994.
Fanon, Frantz. *Toward the African Revolution.* 1956. Translated by Haakon Chevalier. Grove Press, 1994.
Fanon, Frantz. *The Wretched of the Earth.* 1961. Translated by Richard Philcox, Grove Press, 2004.

Fanon, Frantz, and Jacques Azoulay. "Social Therapy in a Ward of Muslim Men: Methodological Difficulties." 1954. Translated by Steven Corcoran. *Frantz Fanon, Alienation and Freedom*, edited by Jean Khalfa and Robert J.C. Young. Bloomsbury Academic, 2018, pp. 353–372.

Fendt, Julia. "The Chromosome as Concept and Metaphor in Amitav Ghosh's *The Calcutta Chromosome.*" *Anglia*, vol. 133, no. 1, 2015, pp. 172–186. www.core.ac.uk/download/pdf/326016009.pdf. Accessed 5 Jul. 2023.

Fett, Sharla M. *Working Cures: Healing, Health, and Power on Southern Plantations.* University of North Carolina Press, 2002.

Fields, Sherry. "Pestilence and Headcolds." *Pestilence and Headcolds: Encountering Illness in Colonial Mexico.* Columbia University Press, 2008. www.gutenberg-e.org/fields/chapter1.html. Accessed 27 Mar. 2022.

Fisher, Dexter. "Stories and their Tellers–A Conversation with Leslie Marmon Silko." *The Third Woman: Minority Women Writers of the United States*, edited by Dexter Fisher. Houghton Mifflin, 1980, pp. 18–23.

Flexner, Abraham. *Medical Education: A Comparative Study.* MacMillan, 1925. www.books.google.dz/books/about/Medical_Education.html?id=s-YWAAAAIAAJ&redir_esc=y. Accessed 25 Nov. 2023.

Forbes, Jack D. *Columbus and Other Cannibals: The Wetiko Disease of Exploitation, Imperialism and Terrorism.* 1978. Seven Stories Press, 2008.

Ford, Julian D., et al. "Psychiatric Comorbidity of Developmental Trauma Disorder and Posttraumatic Stress Disorder: Findings from the DTD Field Trial Replication (DTDFT-R)." *European Journal of Psychotraumatology*, vol. 12, no. 1, 2021, pp. 1–16. www.ncbi.nlm.nih.gov/pmc/articles/PMC8245086/pdf/ZEPT_12_1929028.pdf. Accessed 11 Feb. 2023.

Foucault, Michel. *The Birth of the Clinic: An Archaeology of Medical Perception.* 1963. Translated by A. M. Sheridan Smith. Routledge, 2003.

Foucault, Michel. *Power/Knowledge: Selected Interviews and Other Writings.* Translated by Colin Gordon et al., Random House, 1980.

Four Worlds Development Project: The Sacred Tree. University of Lethbridge Press, 1988.

Frank, Arthur. *The Wounded Storyteller: Body, Illness and Ethics.* The University of Chicago Press, 1997.

Frankl, Viktor E. *The Will to Meaning: Foundations and Applications of Logotherapy.* World Publishing Co., 1969.

Garland-Thomson, Rosemarie. *Extraordinary Bodies: Figuring Physical Disability in American Culture and Literature.* Columbia University Press, 1997.

Garland-Thomson, Rosemarie. "Ways of Staring." *Journal of Visual Culture*, vol. 5, no. 2, 2006, pp. 173 192. www.journals.sagepub.com/doi/10.1177/1470412906066907. Accessed 10 Sep. 2022.

Gberie, Lansana. *A Dirty War in West Africa: The RUF and the Destruction of Sierra Leone.* Indiana University Press, 2005.

Ghosh, Amitav. *The Calcutta Chromosome: A Novel of Fevers, Delirium, and Discovery.* 1995. Murray, 2011.

Ghosh, Bishnupriya. "Animating Uncommon Life: U.S. Military Malaria Films (1942–1945) and the Pacific Theater." *Animating Film Theory*, edited by Karen Beckman. Duke University Press, 2014, pp. 264 286.

Glotfelty, Cheryll. "Introduction: Literary Studies in an Age of Environmental Crisis." *The Ecocriticism Reader: Landmarks in Literary Ecology*, edited by Cheryll Glotfelty and Harold Fromm. University of Georgia Press, 1996, pp. xv xxxvii.

Goodley, Dan. *Disability Studies: An Interdisciplinary Introduction.* SAGE, 2011.

Grinde, Bjorn, and Grete G. Patil. "Biophilia: Does Visual Contact with Nature Impact on Health and Well-Being?" *International Journal of Environmental Research and Public Health*, vol. 6, no. 9, 2009, pp. 2332–2343. www.ncbi.nlm.nih.gov/pmc/articles/PMC2760412/. Accessed 23 Aug. 2022.

Grinde, Donald A., and Bruce E. Johansen. *Ecocide of Native America: Environmental Destruction of Indian Lands and Peoples.* Clear Light, 1995.

Guidotti, Tee L. "The Literal Meaning of Health." *Archives of Environmental and Occupational Health*, vol. 66, no. 3, 2011, pp. 189–190. www.tandfonline.com/doi/abs/10.1080/19338244.2011.585096. Accessed 28 Oct. 2022.

Hakemulder, Frank. *The Moral Laboratory: Experiments Examining the Effects of Reading Literature on Social Perception and Moral Self-Concept.* John Benjamins, 2000.

Hall, Alice. *Literature and Disability.* Routledge, 2015.

Harris, David A. "Pathways to Embodied Empathy and Reconciliation after Atrocity: Former Boy Soldiers in a Dance/Movement Therapy Group in Sierra Leone." *Intervention: The International Journal of Mental Health, Psychosocial Work and Counselling in Areas of Armed Conflict*, vol. 5, no. 3, 2007, pp. 203–231. www.interventionjournal.com/sites/default/files/harris.pdf. Accessed 21 Feb. 2023.

Hartmann, Franz. *Occult Science in Medicine.* Theosophical Publishing Society, 1893. www.ia800701.us.archive.org/29/items/occultscienceinm00hart/occultscienceinm00hart.pdf. Accessed 17 May 2023.

Hawkins, Anne H. "Pathography: Patient Narratives of Illness." *Culture and Medicine*, vol. 171, no. 2, 1999, pp. 127–129.

Head, Bessie. *A Question of Power.* Heinemann, 1973.

Henke, Suzette. *Shattered Subjects: Trauma and Testimony in Women's Life-Writing.* St. Martin's, 1999.

"HIV and AIDS." World Health Organization. Latest update 19 Apr. 2023. www.who.int/news-room/fact-sheets/detail/hiv-aids. Accessed 3 Dec. 2022.

Hirsch, Marianne. "The Generation of Postmemory." *Poetics Today*, vol. 29, no. 1, 2008, pp. 103–128. www.historiaeaudiovisual.weebly.com/uploads/1/7/7/4/17746215/hirsch_postmemory.pdf. Accessed 1 Jul. 2022.

Hogan, Andrew J. "Social and Medical Models of Disability and Mental Health: Evolution and Renewal." *Canadian Medical Association Journal*, vol. 191, no. 1, 2019, pp. E16–E18. www.ncbi.nlm.nih.gov/pmc/articles/PMC6312522/pdf/1910e16.pdf. Accessed 25 Jan. 2022.

Hogan, Linda. *Dwellings.* Touchstone, 1996.

Hooker, Claire, et al. "Health and Medical Humanities in Global Health: From the Anglocentric to the Anthropocene." *Handbook of Social Sciences and Global Public Health*, edited by Pranee Liamputtong. Springer, 2023, pp. 203–220.

Houser, Heather. *Ecosickness in Contemporary U.S. Fiction: Environment and Affect.* Columbia University Press, 2014.

Howe, George. "An Applied Literature." *Studies in Philology*, vol. 17, no. 4, 1920, pp. 423–438. www.archive.org/stream/studiesinphilolo17nortuoft/studiesinphilolo17nortuoft_djvu.txt. Accessed 12 Aug. 2015.

Hudson, Peter. "The State and the Colonial Unconscious." *Social Dynamics*, vol. 39, no. 2, 2013, pp. 263–277. www.tandfonline.com/doi/abs/10.1080/02533952.2013.802867. Accessed 14 Feb. 2023.

Hunt, Paul. *Stigma: The Experience of Disability.* Chapman, 1966.

Jarrett-Macauley, Delia. *Moses, Citizen and Me.* Granta Books, 2005.

Jones, Esther L. *Medicine and Ethics in Black Women's Speculative Fiction*. Palgrave Macmillan, 2015.
Katju, Justice M. "The Truth about Pakistan." *The Nation*. 2 Mar. 2013, p. 7. www.nation.com.pk/pakistan-news-newspaper-daily-english-online/columns/02-Mar-2013/the-truth-about-pakistan. Accessed 12 Oct. 2022.
Khalikova, Venera. "Medical Pluralism." *The Open Encyclopedia of Anthropology*, edited by Felix Stein, 2021. www.anthroencyclopedia.com/printpdf/1471. Accessed 17 Jul. 2023.
Klasen, Fionna, et al. "Posttraumatic Resilience in Former Ugandan Child Soldiers." *Child Development*, vol. 81, no. 4, 2010, pp. 1096–1113. www.pubmed.ncbi.nlm.nih.gov/20636684/. Accessed 10 Nov. 2013.
Klugman, Craig M., and Erin G. Lamb. "Introduction: Raising Health Humanities." *Research Methods in Health Humanities*, edited by Craig M. Klugman and Erin G. Lamb. Oxford University Press, 2019, pp. 1–11.
Koch, Alexander, et al. "Earth System Impacts of the European Arrival and Great Dying in the Americas after 1492." *Quaternary Science Reviews*, vol. 207, 2019, pp. 13–36. www.sciencedirect.com/science/article/pii/S0277379118307261. Accessed 26 Nov. 2023.
Koplan, Jeffrey P., et al. "Towards a Common Definition of Global Health." *Lancet*, vol. 373, no. 9679, 2009, pp. 1993–1995. www.pubmed.ncbi.nlm.nih.gov/19493564/. Accessed 30 May 2023.
Kriegel, Leonard. "The Cripple in Literature." *Images of the Disabled/Disabling Images*, edited by Alan Gartner and Tom Joe. Praeger, 1987, pp. 31–46.
Kutler, Stanley I., ed. *Dictionary of American History* 3rd ed. Gale Group, 2003.
Kwete, Xiaoxiao, et al. "Decolonizing Global Health: What Should Be the Target of this Movement and Where Does it Lead us?" *Global Health Research and Policy*, vol. 7, no. 1, 2022. www.ghrp.biomedcentral.com/articles/10.1186/s41256-022-00237-3. Accessed 5 Jul. 2023.
LaCapra, Dominick. *Writing History, Writing Trauma*. Hopkins University Press, 2001.
LaDuke, Winona. *All Our Relations: Native Struggles for Land Rights and Life*. South End Press, 1999.
Laing, Ronald D. *The Divided Self: An Existential Study in Sanity and Madness*. Penguin, 1990.
Laporte, Dominique. *History of Shit*. MIT Press, 2000.
Lawrence, Jeffrey. "The Global Anglophone: An Institutional Argument." *Interventions: International Journal of Postcolonial Studies*, 0.0, 2023 www.tandfonline.com/doi/epdf/10.1080/1369801X.2022.2161056?needAccess=true&role=button. Accessed 26 May 2023.
Levinas, Emmanuel. *Totality and Infinity: An Essay on Exteriority*. 1969. Translated by Alphonso Lingis. Duquesne University Press, 2002.
Louv, Richard. *Last Child in the Woods: Saving our Children from Nature-Deficit Disorder*. Algonquin Books, 2005.
Lowe, Lisa, and Kris Manjapra. "Comparative Global Humanities after Man: Alternatives to the Coloniality of Knowledge." *Theory, Culture and Society*, vol. 36, no. 5, 2019, pp. 23–48. www.journals.sagepub.com/doi/abs/10.1177/0263276419854795. Accessed 10 Nov. 2023.
Lyotard, Jean-Francois. *The Postmodern Condition: A Report on Knowledge*. Translated by Geoff Bennington and Brian Massumi. University of Minnesota Press, 1984.
MacIntyre, Alasdair. *After Virtue: A Study in Moral Theory*. University of Notre Dame, 1981.
Macnaughton, Jane. "The Humanities in Medical Education: Context, Outcomes and Structures." *Journal of Medical Ethics: Medical Humanities*, vol. 26, no. 1, 2000, pp. 23–30. www.pubmed.ncbi.nlm.nih.gov/12484317/. Accessed 21 Jul. 2022.
Macnaughton, Jane. "Medical Humanities' Challenge to Medicine." *Journal of Evaluation in Clinical Practice*, vol. 17, no. 5, 2011, pp. 927–932. www.pubmed.ncbi.nlm.nih.gov/21851510/. Accessed 21 Jul. 2022.

Mandova, Evans. "The Shona Proverb as an Expression of Unhu/Ubuntu." *Matatu*, vol. 41, no. 1, 2013, pp. 357–368. www.proquest.com/docview/1449638827. Accessed 25 May 2022.

Marinker, Marshall. "Why Make People Patients?" *Journal of Medical Ethics*, vol. 1, no. 2, 1975, pp. 81–84. www.ncbi.nlm.nih.gov/pmc/articles/PMC1154460/. Accessed 23 Dec. 2022.

Marks, Deborah. *Disability: Controversial Debates and Psychosocial Perspectives*. Taylor & Frances/Routledge, 1999.

Marx, Christopher, et al. "Talking Cure Models: A Framework of Analysis." *Frontiers in Psychology*, vol. 8, art. 1589, 2017, pp. 1–13. www.ncbi.nlm.nih.gov/pmc/articles/PMC5601393/pdf/fpsyg-08-01589.pdf. Accessed 11 Jan. 2022.

Maslow, Abraham H. *Motivation and Personality*. 1954. Harper & Row, 1970.

Masterson, John. *John Mordaunt: Facing up to AIDS, as Told to John Masterson*. O'Brien Press, 1989.

McLellan, M. Faith. "Literature and Medicine: Narratives of Physical Illness." The Lancet, vol. 349, no. 9065, 1997, pp. 1618–1620. www.thelancet.com/pdfs/journals/lancet/PIIS0140-6736(97)04429-2.pdf. Accessed 8 Dec. 2022.

Meade, Erica H. *Tell it by Heart: Women and the Healing Power of Story*. Open Court, 1995.

Meekosha, Helen. "Decolonising Disability: Thinking and Acting Globally." *Disability and Society*, vol. 26, no. 6, 2011, pp. 667–682. www.tandfonline.com/doi/abs/10.1080/09687599.2011.602860. Accessed 8 Dec. 2022.

Mersmann, Birgit, and Hans G. Kippenberg. *The Humanities between Global Integration and Cultural Diversity*. De Gruyter, 2016.

Mitchell, David T., and Sharon L. Snyder. *Narrative Prosthesis: Disability and the Dependencies of Discourse*. University of Michigan Press, 2000.

Modaff, Daniel P. "*Mitakuye Oyasin* (We Are All Related)." *Great Plains Quarterly*, vol. 39, no. 4, 2019, pp. 341–362. www.jstor.org/stable/26827321. Accessed 2 Nov. 2021.

Morrison, Toni. *Jazz*. Knopf, 1992.

Morrison, Toni. *A Mercy*. Knopf, 2008.

Murray, Stuart. "From Virginia's Sister to Friday's Silence: Presence, Metaphor, and the Persistence of Disability in Contemporary Writing." *Journal of Literary and Cultural Disability Studies*, vol. 6, no. 3, 2012, pp. 241–258. www.muse.jhu.edu/article/487892/pdf. Accessed 2 Nov. 2021.

Mwangi, Meja. *Crossroads: The Last Plague*. 1997. HM Books, 2008.

"Multiculturalism." *The Canadian Encyclopedia*. www.thecanadianencyclopedia.ca/en/article/multiculturalism. Accessed 10 Sep. 2022.

Nair, Supriya. "Melancholic Women: The Intellectual Hysteric(s) in *Nervous Conditions*." *Research in African Literatures*, vol. 26, no. 2, 1995, pp. 130–139. www.jstor.org/stable/3820276. Accessed 12 Sep. 2019.

Nario-Redmond, Michelle R., et al. "Hostile, Benevolent, and Ambivalent Ableism: Contemporary Manifestations." *Journal of Social Issues*, vol. 75, no. 3, 2019, pp. 726–756. www.spssi.onlinelibrary.wiley.com/doi/10.1111/josi.12337. Accessed 20 Jul. 2022.

Nash, Woods. "Showing that Medical Ethics Cases Can Miss the Point: Rewriting Short Stories as Cases." *Literature and Medicine*, vol. 36, no. 1, 2018, pp. 190–207. www.muse.jhu.edu/article/698167/pdf. Accessed 7 Nov. 2023.

"Native Americans' Many Contributions to Medicine." US Embassy and Consulates in Italy 18 Nov. 2021. www.it.usembassy.gov/native-americans-many-contributions-to-medicine/. Accessed 15 Mar. 2022.

Newell, Stephanie. "Conflict and Transformation in Bessie Head's *A Question of Power, Serowe: Village of the Rain Wind* and *A Bewitched Crossroad.*" *The Journal of Commonwealth Literature*, vol. 30 no. 2, 1995, pp. 65–83.

Nott, Josiah C., and George R. Gliddon. *Indigenous Races of the Earth; or, New Chapters of Ethnological Inquiry; Including Monographs on Special Departments.* Lippincott & Co., 1857. www.archive.org/details/cu31924029883752. Accessed 7 Jul. 2022.

Nunn, Nathan, and Nancy Qian. "The Columbian Exchange: A History of Disease, Food, and Ideas." *Journal of Economic Perspectives*, vol. 24, no. 2, 2010, pp. 163–188. www.pubs.aeaweb.org/doi/pdfplus/10.1257/jep.24.2.163. Accessed 25 May 2022.

Olkin, Rhoda. *What Psychotherapists Should Know about Disability.* Guilford Press, 1999.

Osler, William. *Aequanimitas, with other Addresses to Medical Students, Nurses and Practitioners of Medicine.* P. Blakiston's Son & Co., 1904. www.babel.hathitrust.org/cgi/pt?id=aeu.ark:/13960/t3xs7cx3p&seq=1. Accessed 2 Aug. 2021.

Osler, William. "The Old Humanities and the New Science." *British Medical Journal*, vol. 2, no. 3053, 1919, pp. 1–7. www.ncbi.nlm.nih.gov/pmc/articles/PMC2343167/pdf/brmedj07003-0027.pdf. Accessed 2 May 2022.

Packard, Randall M. *The Making of a Tropical Disease: A Short History of Malaria.* The Johns Hopkins University Press, 2007.

Pailey, Robtel N. "An Interview with Tsitsi Dangarembga." *Pambazuka News.* 5 Oct. 2006. www.pambazuka.org/arts/interview-tsitsi-dangarembga. Accessed 11 Nov. 2022.

Pearse, Adetokunbo. "Apartheid and Madness: Bessie Head's *A Question of Power.*" *Kunapipi*, vol. 5, no. 2, 1983, pp. 81–98.

Peiretti-Courtis, Delphine. "The Construction of Racial Knowledge by Colonial Medicine in Africa." *Encyclopédie d'histoire numérique de l'Europe.* Sorbonne Université, 2022. www.ehne.fr/en/node/21439/printable/pdf. Accessed 11 Jan. 2023

Perez Foster, Rose Mary "When Immigration is Trauma: Guidelines for the Individual and Family Clinician." *The American Journal of Orthopsychiatry*, vol. 71, no. 2, 2001, pp. 153–170. www.sjsu.edu/people/edward.cohen/courses/c3/s1/immigration_trauma.pdf. Accessed 10 Jan. 2023.

Platt, Frederic W. "Clinical Hypocompetence: The Interview." *Annals of Internal Medicine*, no. 91, 1979, pp. 898–902.

Poskett, James. "Phrenology, Correspondence, and the Global Politics of Reform, 1815–1848." *The Historical Journal*, vol. 60, no. 2, 2017, pp. 409–442. www.wrap.warwick.ac.uk/101955/. Accessed 10 Nov. 2022.

Powell, John W. *Seventh Annual Report of the Bureau of Ethnology.* Government Printing Office, 1891. www.gutenberg.org/files/26568/26568-h/26568-h.htm. Accessed 16 Jan. 2022.

Quayson, Ato. *Aesthetic Nervousness: Disability and the Crisis of Representation.* Columbia University Press, 2007.

Quinlan, Marsha B. "Ethnomedicine." *A Companion of Medical Anthropology*, edited by Merrill Singer and Pamela I. Erickson. Blackwell, 2011, pp. 381–403.

Rabelais, François. *Pantagruel.* Maison de Claude Nourry, 1532. http://www.coillet.eu/Site/Documents/Pantagruel.pdf

Ramjee, Gita, and Brodie Daniels. "Women and HIV in Sub-Saharan Africa." *AIDS Research and Therapy*, vol. 10, no. 30, 2013, pp. 1–9. www.aidsrestherapy.biomedcentral.com/articles/10.1186/1742-6405-10-30. Accessed 12 Jan. 2023.

Ranlet, Phillip. "The British, the Indians, and Smallpox: What Actually Happened at Fort Pitt in 1763?" *Pennsylvania History*, vol. 67, no. 3, 2000, pp. 427–441. www.jstor.org/stable/27774278. Accessed 10 Jul. 2010.

Richards, Paul. *Fighting for the Rain Forest: War, Youth and Resources in Sierra Leone*. James Currey, 1996.

Roberts, Dorothy. *Fatal Invention: How Science, Politics, and Big Business Re-Create Race in the Twenty-First Century*. New Press, 2011.

Rose, Arthur. "Mood, Health, and the Global Anglophone." *Post45: Forms of the Global Anglophone*, 2019. www.post45.org/2019/02/mood-health-and-the-global-anglophone-novel/. Accessed 25 May 2023.

Rosen, David M. "Child Soldiers, International Humanitarian Law, and the Globalization of Childhood." *American Anthropologist*, vol. 109, no. 2, 2007, pp. 296–306. www.jstor.org/stable/4496643. Accessed 20 Dec. 2013.

Ross, Ronald. "The Malaria Expedition in West Africa." *Science*, vol. 11, no. 262, 1900, pp. 36–37. www.science.org/doi/10.1126/science.11.262.36. Accessed 2 Dec. 2022.

Ross, Ronald. *Memoirs: With a Full Account of the Great Malaria Problem and its Solution*. John Murray, 1923. www.wellcomecollection.org/works/ckfaqbds/items. Accessed 2 Dec. 2022.

Roszak, Theodore. "Awakening the Ecological Unconscious." *Context*, vol. 34, 1993, pp. 48–51.

Roy, Animesh. "From the Clinical to the Ecocultural: Literature, Health, and Ethnoecomedicine." *The Bloomsbury Handbook to Medical-Environmental Humanities*, edited by Scott Slovic, et al. Bloomsbury Academic Press, 2022, pp. 251–260.

Rushdie, Salman. *Shame*. Vintage, 1995.

Rust, Mary-Jayne. "Forward." *Environmental Arts Therapy: The Wild Frontiers of the Heart*, edited by Ian Siddons Heginworth and Gary Nash. Routledge, 2020.

Rutten, Anja X., et al. "Autism in Adult and Juvenile Delinquents: A Literature Review." *Child Adolescent and Psychiatry and Mental Health*, vol. 11, no. 45, 2017, pp. 1–12. www.capmh.biomedcentral.com/articles/10.1186/s13034-017-0181-4. Accessed 25 Sep. 2022.

Sacks, Oliver W. *The Man who Mistook his Wife for a Hat and Other Clinical Tales*. Summit Books, 1985.

Sacks, Oliver W. "Sacks to Luria." 14 June 1975, Oliver Sacks Archives, Oliver Sacks Foundation, New York City.

Sandner, Donald. *Navaho Symbols of Healing: A Jungian Exploration of Ritual, Image & Medicine*. 1979. Healing Arts Press, 1991.

Sarton, George, and Frances Siegel. "Seventy-First Critical Bibliography of the History and Philosophy of Science and of the History of Civilization (to October 1947)." *Isis*, vol. 39, no. 1/2, 1948, pp. 70–139. www.jstor.org/stable/226775. Accessed 15 Nov. 2022.

Sartre, Jean-Paul. "Preface." *The Wretched of the Earth*. 1961. Translated by Richard Philcox, Grove Press, 2004, pp. xIii–lxii.

Schauer, Maggie, et al. *Narrative Exposure Therapy: A Short-Term Intervention for Traumatic Stress Disorders after War, Terror, or Torture*. Hogrefe, 2005.

Sekyi-Out, Ato. *Fanon's Dialectic of Experience*. Harvard University Press, 1996.

Shakespeare, Tom, et al. *The Sexual Politics of Disability: Untold Desires*. Cassell, 1996.

Shiva, Vandana. "Women, Ecology and Health: Rebuilding Connections." *Close to Home: Women Reconnect Ecology, Health and Development*, edited by Vandana Shiva. Earthscan, 1994, pp. 1–9.

Sidhwa, Bapsi. *Cracking India: A Novel*. Milkweed Editions, 1991.

Siebers, Tobin. *Disability Theory*. University of Michigan Press, 2008.

Silko, Leslie M. *Ceremony*. Penguin Books, 1977.

Silko, Leslie M. *Yellow Woman and a Beauty of the Spirit: Essays on Native American Life Today.* Touchstone, 1996.

Slovic, Scott, et al. "Introduction: Toward a Medical-Environmental Humanities: Why Now?" *The Bloomsbury Handbook to Medical-Environmental Humanities*, edited by Scott Slovic, et al. Bloomsbury Academic Press, 2022, pp. 1–10.

Smith, Michael K. *The Greatest Story Never Told: A People's History of the American Empire, 1945–1999.* Xlibris Corporation, 2001.

Snow, Charles P. *The Two Cultures.* 1959. *Leonardo*, vol. 2, no. 3, 1990, pp. 169–173. www.sciencepolicy.colorado.edu/students/envs_5110/snow_1959.pdf. Accessed 25 Dec. 2022.

Snyder, Sharon L., and David T. Mitchell. *Cultural Locations of Disability.* University of Chicago Press, 2006.

Snyder, Sharon L., and David T. Mitchell. "Disability Haunting in American Poetics." *The Journal of Literary Disability*, vol. 1, no. 1, 2007, pp. 1–12. www.liverpooluniversitypress.co.uk/doi/10.3828/jlcds.1.1.2. Accessed 10 Nov. 2022.

Sontag, Susan. *AIDS and its Metaphors.* Farrar, Straus and Giroux, 1989.

Sontag, Susan. *Illness as Metaphor.* Farrar, Straus and Giroux, 1978.

Spivak, Gayatri C. "Can the Subaltern Speak?" *Marxism and the Interpretation of Culture*, edited by Nelson Carry and Lawrence Grossberg. University of Illinois Press, 1988, pp. 271–313.

Srinivasan, Ragini T. "Introduction: South Asia from Postcolonial to World Anglophone." *Interventions: International Journal of Postcolonial Studies*, vol. 20, no. 3, 2018, pp. 309–316. www.tandfonline.com/doi/abs/10.1080/1369801X.2018.1446840. Accessed 25 May 2025.

Steinberg, Erwin R. "Applied Humanities?" *College English*, vol. 35, no. 4, 1974, pp. 440–450.

Stewart, Kearsley A., and Kelley K. Swain. "Global Health Humanities: Defining an Emerging Field." *The Lancet*, no. 388, 2016, pp. 2586–2587. www.thelancet.com/journals/lancet/issue/vol388no10060/PIIS0140-6736(16)X0051-7. Accessed 5 Aug. 2022.

Szasz, Thomas S., and Marc H. Hollender. "A Contribution to the Philosophy of Medicine; the Basic Models of the Doctor-Patient Relationship." *A.M.A. Archives of Internal Medicine*, vol. 97, no. 5, 1956, pp. 585–592. www.pubmed.ncbi.nlm.nih.gov/13312700/. Accessed 3 Jan. 2023.

Talahite, Anissa. "Cape Gooseberries and Giant Cauliflowers: Transplantation, Hybridity and Growth in Bessie Head's *A Question of Power.*" *Mosaic*, vol. 38, no. 4, 2005, pp. 141–157. www.jstor.org/stable/44030091. Accessed 5 Nov. 2021.

Todd, Jude. "Knotted Bellies and Fragile Webs: Untangling and Re-Spinning in Tayo's Healing Journey." *American Indian Quarterly*, vol. 19, no. 2, 1995, pp. 155–170.

Trans-continental Tourist's Guide. Geo. A. Crofutt, c1872. www.library.si.edu/digital-library/book/crofuttstranscon00newy. Accessed 30 Jan. 2023.

Tsampiras Carla, and Alex Müller. "Overcoming 'Minimal Objectivity' and 'Inherent Bias': Ethics and Understandings of Feminist Research in a Health Sciences Faculty in South Africa." *Feminist Encounters: A Journal of Critical Studies in Culture and Politics*, vol. 2, no. 2, 2018, pp. 1–16. www.lectitopublishing.nl/download/overcoming-minimal-objectivity-and-inherent-bias-ethics-and-understandings-of-feminist-research-in-a-3884.pdf. Accessed 10 Jan. 2022.

Turner, Victor W. *The Ritual Process: Structure and Anti-structure.* Aldine Publishing Co., 1969.

Turner, Victor W. *From Ritual to Theatre: The Human Seriousness of Play.* PAJ Publications, 1982.

Ulrich, Roger S. "Effects of Gardens on Health Outcomes: Theory and Research." *Healing Gardens Therapeutic Benefits and Design Recommendations*, edited by Marcus C. Cooper and Marni Barnes. John Wiley & Sons, 1999, pp. 27–86.

Ulrich, Roger S. "View through a Window may Influence Recovery." *Science*, vol. 224, no. 4647, 1984, pp. 224–225. www.pubmed.ncbi.nlm.nih.gov/6143402/. Accessed 16 May 2023.

UNCRDP. "Convention on the Rights of Persons with Disabilities and Optional Protocol." United Nations, 2006. www.un.org/disabilities/documents/convention/convoptprot-e.pdf. Accessed 12 Nov. 2022.

Union of the Physically Impaired against Segregation and Disability Alliance. "Fundamental Principles of Disability." 1977. www.disability-studies.leeds.ac.uk/wp-content/uploads/sites/40/library/UPIAS-fundamental-principles.pdf. Accessed 11 Jan. 2022.

United Nations. "The 17 Goals." www.sdgs.un.org/fr/goals. Accessed 12 Dec. 2021.

Van der Kolk, Bassel A. "The Complexity of Adaptation to Trauma: Self-regulation, Stimulus Discrimination, and Characterological Development." *Traumatic Stress: The Effects of Overwhelming Experience on Mind, Body, and Society*, edited by Bassel A. Van der Kolk, et al. The Guilford Press, 1996, pp. 182–213.

Van der Kolk, Bessel A., and Onno van der Hart. "The Intrusive Past: The Flexibility of Memory and the Engraving of Trauma." *Trauma: Explorations in Memory*, edited by Cathy Caruth. Johns Hopkins, 1995, pp. 158–182.

Visser, Irene. "Decolonizing Trauma Theory: Retrospect and Prospects." *Humanities*, vol. 4, no. 2, 2015, pp. 250–265. www.mdpi.com/2076–0787/4/2/250. Accessed 2 Nov. 2021.

Visser, Irene. "Trauma Theory and Postcolonial Literary Studies." *Journal of Postcolonial Writing*, vol. 47, no. 3, 2011, pp. 270–282. www.tandfonline.com/doi/abs/10.1080/17449855.2011.569378. Accessed 2 Nov. 2021.

Vizenor, Gerald. *Fugitive Poses: Native American Indian Scenes of Absence and Presence*. University of Nebraska Press, 1998.

Vizenor, Gerald. *Manifest Manners: Postindian Warriors of Survivance*. Wesleyan/New England University Press, 1994.

Vogel, Virgil J. "American Indian Influence on the American Pharmacopeia." *American Indian Culture and Research Journal*, vol. 2, no. 1, 1977, pp. 3–7. www.eric.ed.gov/?id=ED138390. Accessed 12 Dec. 2021.

Walton, Samantha. "Eco-Recovery Memoir and the Medical-Environmental Humanities." *The Routledge Companion to Health Humanities*, edited by Paul Crawford, et al. Routledge, 2020, pp. 97–113.

Wailoo, Keith. "Patients Are Humans Too: The Emergence of Medical Humanities." *Daedalus*, vol. 151, no. 3, 2022, pp. 194–205. www.jstor.org/stable/48681153. Accessed 29 Jul. 2022.

Warren, Karen J. *Ecofeminist Philosophy: A Western Perspective on what it Is and why it Matters*. Rowman & Littlefield Publishers, 2000.

Washington, Harriet A. *Medical Apartheid: The Dark History of Medical Experimentation on Black Americans from Colonial Times to the Present*. Anchor, 2006.

Wernli, Didier, et al. "Moving Global Health Forward in Academic Institutions." *Journal of Global Health*, vol. 6, no. 1, 2016, p. 010409. www.ncbi.nlm.nih.gov/pmc/articles/PMC4766794/. Accessed 16 Sep. 2022.

Wesley-Esquimaux, Cynthia, and Magdalena Smolewski. *Historic Trauma and Aboriginal Healing*. Aboriginal Healing Foundation, 2004.

West, Jessamyn. *To See the Dream*. Harcourt, Brace & Company, 1957.

Whitehead, Anne. "Representing the Child Solider: Trauma, Postcolonialism and Ethics in Delia Jarrett-Macauley's *Moses, Citizen and Me*." *Ethics and Trauma in Contemporary British Fiction*, edited by Susana Onega, et al. Rodopi Press, 2011, pp. 243–263.

Whiteley, Paul, et al. "Autoimmune Encephalitis and Autism Spectrum Disorder." *Frontiers in Psychiatry*, vol. 12, Article 775017, 2021, pp. 1–9. www.frontiersin.org/articles/10.3389/fpsyt.2021.775017. Accessed 9 Nov. 2022.

Williamson, John. "The Disarmament, Demobilization and Reintegration of Child Soldiers: Social and Psychological Transformation in Sierra Leone." *Intervention*, vol. 4, no. 3, 2006, pp. 185–205. www.semanticscholar.org/paper/The-disarmament%2C-demobilization-and-reintegration-Williamson/5bbd787a17c6bb1d4f340374ebf02b6d48ae92d8. Accessed 2 Sep. 2013.

Wilson, Margon, and Martin Daly. "Competitiveness, Risk Taking, and Violence: The Young Male Syndrome." *Ethnology and Sociobiology*, no. 6, 1985, pp. 59–73. www.martindaly.ca/uploads/2/3/7/0/23707972/wilson__daly_1985_young_male_syndrome.pdf. Accessed 12 Nov. 2022.

Wolff, Ilze. "The Garden as a Site of Colonial Critique." *The Architectural Review*. 19 Oct. 2020. www.architectural-review.com/essays/home-ground-the-garden-as-a-site-of-colonial-critique. Accessed 21 Dec. 2022.

World Health Organization (WHO). *Promoting Mental Health: Concepts, Emerging Evidence, Practice: A Report of the World Health Organization*. 1 Jan. 2005. www.who.int/publications/i/item/9241562943. Accessed 28 Sep. 2022.

World Health Organization (WHO). "Traditional Medicine, Fact Sheet No. 134." 2003. www.who.int/mediacentre/factsheets/fs 134/en/. Accessed 28 Sep. 2020.

Wyatt, Jean. "Failed Messages, Maternal Loss, and Narrative Form in Toni Morrison's *A Mercy*." *Modern Fiction Studies*, vol. 58, no. 1, 2012, pp. 128–151. www.muse.jhu.edu/article/470664/pdf. Accessed 20 Nov. 2021.

Zamora, Lois P. "Magical Romance/Magical Realism: Ghosts in U.S. and Latin American Fiction." *Magical Realism: Theory, History, Community*, edited by Lois P. Zamora and Wendy B. Faris. Duke University Press, 1995, pp. 497–550.

Index of Persons

Anderson, Warwick   21
Ashcroft, Bill   6, 45

Barker, Clare   53 f., 115 f.
Benatar, Solomon   18
Bleakley, Alan   25
Boehmer, Elleke   46
Brave Heart, Maria Y. H.   31, 63
Brison, Susan J.   107
Brody, Howard   4, 29

Campbell, Fiona K.   121, 129
Chariandy, David   12, 104, 106–110, 165
Charon, Rita   42 f.
Coetzee, J.M.   12, 125, 127–133, 165
Cole, Thomas R.   27, 101
Craps, Stef   47
Crawford, Allison   32
Crawford, Paul   VI, 4, 8, 24, 29
Crosby, Alfred W.   59 f.

Dangarembga, Tsitsi   12, 53, 92, 94–99, 101, 103, 164
Darian-Smith, Eve   4 f.
DasGupta, Sayantani   20
Davis, Lennard J.   50 f.
DeBruyn, Lemyra M.   63
Dudley, Rachel   37

Engel, George L.   26 f.
Erdrich, Louise   11, 59, 61, 63 f., 164

Fanon, Frantz   11, 23–25, 47, 76, 92–94, 97–100, 103, 147, 163
Foucault, Michel   68, 71, 94, 130

Ghosh, Amitav   11, 66–72, 164
Glotfelty, Cheryll   7

Hawkins, Anne H.   52, 137
Head, Bessie   13, 80, 137 f., 140–142, 165
Hirsch, Marianne   109 f.

Jarrett-Macauley, Delia   13, 153 f., 156–161, 166

Koplan, Jeffrey P.   19
Kriegel, Leonard   51
Kwete, Xiaoxiao   25

Silko, Leslie M.   13, 143–148, 150–152, 165
Lawrence, Jeffrey   7, 23, 122

Macnaughton, Jane   4, 29
Maslow, Abraham H.   131
McCarthy, Philip C.   4 f.
Mitchell, David T.   12, 50, 53 f., 113, 119 f., 123, 127, 149, 165
Morrison, Toni   11, 51, 53 f., 85–87, 89–91, 164
Mwangi, Meja   11, 73 f., 76, 78, 81, 164

Osler, William   2

Perez Foster, Rose Mary   105 f.

Quayson, Ato   12, 51 f., 113, 115 f., 119 f., 122, 124–129, 133, 165

Ross, Ronald   66–70, 164
Rushdie, Salman   12, 53, 120–126, 165

Sacks, Oliver W.   40, 44
Sartre, Jean-Paul   92, 99
Shakespeare, Tom   52, 122, 158
Sidhwa, Bapsi   12, 52 f., 113, 115–119, 165
Slovic, Scott   36
Smolewski, Magdalena   32, 63
Snow, Charles P.   2
Snyder, Sharon L.   12, 50, 53 f., 113, 119 f., 123, 127, 165
Sontag, Susan   48
Stewart, Kearsley A.   4, 167
Swain, Kelley K.   4, 167

Turner, Victor W.   160

Ulrich, Roger S.   34 f., 140

Van der Kolk, Bassel A. 87, 155
Visser, Irene 147, 153

Wesley-Esquimaux, Cynthia 32, 63

Index of Subjects

Ableism   12, 38, 50, 120 f., 123 f., 127 – 129
Aesthetic nervousness   12, 51, 53, 123 – 125, 127, 133, 165
AIDS   4, 11, 25, 29 – 30, 48, 73, 75, 77 – 79, 81, 137, 164
Alienation   94, 96, 99, 105 f., 156
Anorexia nervosa   96 f., 101, 164
Applied humanities   2
Applied literature   2, 7 f., 10, 13, 163
Arts therapy   166
Autism   123, 125

Biomedicine   13, 26, 31, 33 f., 38, 166
Biophilia   139
Biopsychosocial   26 – 27, 50, 127
Body   1, 12, 22, 26, 28, 33, 35, 42, 44 – 51, 53, 60, 68, 86, 89, 92, 94 – 96, 98, 100 – 103, 105 f., 108, 117 f., 120, 123, 128, 130 – 132, 145 f., 148, 159 f., 164 f.
boy soldier   13, 153 – 162, 166
Bulimia   95, 101, 164

Class   3, 6, 9 f., 17, 19, 30, 36 – 39, 51 – 54, 92, 96 f., 113, 128 f., 163, 168
Clinical tales   44
Close reading   9, 43, 163
Colonial   5 – 7, 10 f., 19 – 25, 46, 48, 56, 62 f., 69, 72, 85, 92 – 99, 101, 107, 113 – 115, 118 f., 127, 138, 147, 163 f.
Colonial medicine   17, 22 f., 25, 66
Columbian exchange   59
Communitas   13, 160, 162
Corpo-reality   45, 47, 117, 168

Dance therapy   95, 102, 153, 156, 158
Decolonizing   10, 19, 26
Disabled   37, 49 – 50, 53, 115, 122, 126, 129 – 130, 164 – 165, 168
Disease   1, 3, 8 – 11, 13, 19 f., 23 – 26, 28 – 34, 39 f., 42, 44 f., 48 f., 56, 59 – 64, 70, 73 f., 78 f., 81, 97, 108, 113 f., 119, 123, 130, 137 – 139, 144, 148, 156, 163 f., 166 f.

Diversity   5, 17 f., 27, 32, 35, 54, 66, 140, 159, 166
Doctor-patient relationship   133

Eating disorder   12, 94 f., 97, 101, 164
Eco-artistic   13, 153, 156 f., 161 f., 165 – 167
Ecocriticism   6
Ecofeminism   6
Ecological imperialism   60
Ecological unconscious   156
Eco-recovery   143, 147, 157
Ecosickness   148
Empathy   1 f., 9, 18, 26 f., 29, 39 – 41, 54, 56, 96, 100 f., 110, 116, 124, 133, 137 f., 167 f.
Environmental health humanities   13, 163, 168
Environmental humanities   36
Ethical   5, 8, 28, 37, 41, 43 – 45, 130, 133, 168
Ethnomedicine   31, 33 – 35, 38, 166

Feminist Health Humanities   37
Freedom   20, 24, 64, 88, 95, 97, 104, 159

Garden   13, 137, 139 – 141, 165, 167
Gender   3, 6, 9 f., 12, 17, 19, 30, 36 – 39, 51, 53 f., 63, 75 f., 79, 92, 101, 113, 118, 143, 163 f., 167 f.
Global anglophone   1, 3 f., 6 – 13, 17, 19, 34, 39, 42, 45 f., 56, 127, 153, 163, 166 – 168
Global health   1, 3 f., 8 – 10, 13, 17 – 19, 23, 25 f., 38, 45, 56, 69, 73, 75, 163 – 165, 167
Global health humanities   1 – 4, 6, 8 – 11, 13, 17, 19, 25, 30 f., 37 – 39, 56, 73, 163, 165 – 168
Global turn   5 – 7

Health humanities   1, 3 f., 8, 10, 17, 23 f., 27 – 30, 32, 37 – 39, 45, 80, 168
Historical trauma response   31
Historical unresolved grief   59
Holistic healing   3, 10, 13, 34, 146, 165 f.
Horticulture   139

Illness   8, 24, 26 f., 30 f., 43, 48 f., 62, 81, 97, 107, 130, 137, 144 – 147, 149 f., 152
Imperial   5 f., 11, 23, 59, 95, 164

Inclusivity   1, 3–7, 10, 13, 17, 25, 30 f., 38 f., 47, 55 f., 116, 148, 163–165, 168
Indigenous health humanities   31 f.
Infectious disease   48, 74, 77, 89
Intersectionality   17, 19, 36–38, 92, 163, 168

Knowledge systems   11, 18, 66, 68, 71 f.

Life review   73, 78, 80, 132 f.
Literature and medicine   10, 39–41, 44
Logotherapy   42

Madness   24, 68, 88, 106, 137–139, 143
Malaria   11, 59, 66–70, 164
Maternal abandonment   11 f., 85–87, 164
Medical education   3, 25, 27 f., 40, 43, 67
Medical-environmental humanities   36
Medical humanities   3 f., 17, 28–30, 36
Medical model of disability   128
Medical pluralism   35, 66
Mental health   25, 89, 93 f., 106, 137, 139, 141 f., 157, 163, 166
Metaphor   9, 12, 46–48, 52–54, 66, 71, 75, 125, 127, 137, 141, 156, 164 f., 167
Migration   3, 9, 12, 45, 104–110, 164, 167
Moral laboratory   45
Moral model of disability   120, 122
More-than-human   148, 151, 157, 163
Multiculturalism   12, 104

Narrative medicine   42 f., 168
Narrative prosthesis   12, 50, 53, 113, 120, 123, 127, 165
Nature-deficit disorder   156

Occult science   69
One Health   18 f., 163

Pathography   137
Post-colonial   2 f., 5–8, 10–12, 17, 21, 25 f., 30 f., 37, 45–47, 53, 55, 92, 103, 147, 153, 163 f.
Postmemory   19, 31 f., 59, 63, 87 f., 104, 107–110, 146, 155
Presenile dementia   12, 104–110, 164 f.
PTSD   13, 31, 47 f., 143, 145, 165

Ritual   32–34, 52, 69, 143, 145–151, 160

SDG   166 f.
Sickness   8, 43, 48 f., 62–64, 87, 96, 130
Smallpox   59–61, 88 f., 164
Social model of disability   113, 117, 119, 129
Stigma   11 f., 38, 49, 73, 76, 81, 123, 126
storytelling   13, 32–33, 37, 41–42, 45, 64, 143–145, 153, 157, 165–166

Traditional knowledge   17 f., 32 f., 35, 55, 66, 68 f., 71 f., 164
Trauma   2, 10–13, 31, 42, 46–48, 59, 63, 85–87, 89 f., 98, 101, 104–110, 113, 115, 147, 149–151, 153–162, 164–166
Two cultures   2, 97

Unresolved traumatic grief   11, 59, 63 f., 164

Violence   11 f., 71, 85, 91–93, 95, 97 f., 100 f., 105, 107, 113, 115 f., 118 f., 123 f., 127, 153 f., 159, 164, 167
Virgin soil epidemics   11, 59 f., 64, 164

WHO   24, 26, 31, 73